SKIN GRAFTS

Edited by **Madhuri Gore**

Skin Grafts
http://dx.doi.org/10.5772/45962
Edited by Madhuri Gore

Contributors

Joon Pio Hong, Hyunsuk Suh, Thomas Rappl, Yoshiaki Sakamoto, Silvestro Canonico, Ferdinando Campitiello, Angela Della Corte, Vincenzo Padovano, Gianluca Pellino, Rei Ogawa, Anya Li, Tamer Ghanem, Mark Wax, Madhuri Gore

Published by InTech

Janeza Trdine 9, 51000 Rijeka, Croatia

Publishing Process Manager Marija Radja
Technical Editor InTech DTP team
Cover InTech Design team

Additional hard copies can be obtained from orders@intechopen.com

Skin Grafts, Edited by Madhuri Gore
p. cm.
ISBN 978-953-51-0973-0

For EU product safety concerns:
IN TECH d.o.o., Prolaz Marije Krucifikse Kozulić 3, 51000 Rijeka, Croatia,
info@intechopen.com or visit our website at intechopen.com.

Meet the editor

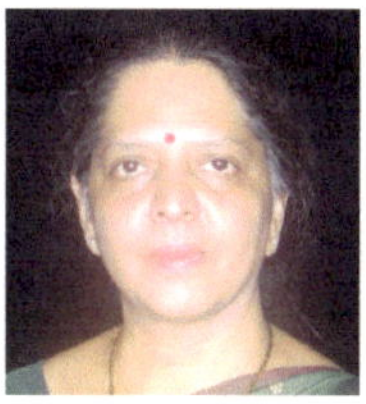

Dr. Gore has been faculty at L T M medical college department of surgery for 30 years and chief of surgery for 11 years. Her fields of interest have been burn and wound care, venous disorders and trauma. As chief of burn care for more than 20 years, she has conducted several research projects, clinical trials and has developed banana leaf dressing and contributed to development of wound care products. Having established the first Allograft Skin bank in India in April 2000 and she introduced the concept of skin donation after death to Indian society. Besides being a sought after speaker, she has contributed more than 50 articles to journals and 8 chapters to different books. Dr. Gore's contribution to training and research in these areas has been acknowledged with awards, orations and felicitations.

Contents

Preface

Split thickness skin grafting procedure is a simple but essential and important one to achieve closure of a full thickness or deep partial thickness skin defect. It needs to be performed with care and precision for successful outcome.

The present publication is devoted to skin grafts. Three important components of this procedure are preparation of wound bed, fixation of skin grafts to the recipient area to improve possibility of graft take and management of skin graft donor area for both full thickness and split thickness grafts. The chapters have been distributed in these three sections.

The preparation of wound bed needs to be optimized so that the take of the graft is ensured. The absence of necrotic tissue, adequacy of vascularisation and absence of infection are the main goals of wound bed preparation. These can be achieved by several means – surgical debridement, enzymatic action, biological methods (maggot therapy) and recently introduced hydro surgery technique using water jet. Negative pressure therapy is becoming popular rapidly as a method of wound improvement. In the presence of wound infection, skin allograft or xenografts can be used effectively to control infection and to improve subsequent allograft take. Skin allograft and xenografts also stimulate epithelisation and thus reduce the area that needs skin auto grafts for wound closure. The section addressing this component has a chapter describing various methods and provides details of hydro surgery equipment and its use for wound debridement.

Ensuring optimal contact of skin grafts with the recipient area is crucial for graft survival. Besides conventional techniques such as staples and suturing, the chapters in this section describe innovative ideas like wire fixation, use of chloramphenical powder for fixing grafts besides the use of negative pressure. For allowing drainage of fluid collected under the graft and for the purpose of expansion of the graft, meshing methods using specific equipments are well known. Here we have an imaginative, simple and cheap method using flower holder. Success of skin grafting procedure contributes significantly to the final outcome in a burnt patient. Evaluation of a standardised skin grafting procedure is the topic of a chapter in this section. The thickness of dermal component varies greatly in a split thickness skin graft. Deficiency of dermis leads to contraction of grafted area and instability as well as compromised cosmetic outcome. Lack of adequate dermal component is probably also responsible for recurrence of chronic ulcers especially venous ulcers. Use of dermal skin substitutes provide this component and allow use of thin auto graft over the neodermis. This strategy is also useful for defects created after release of post burn contracture. In this section we have two chapters describing experience of use of dermal skin substitute on chronic ulcers.

Achieving early healing of skin graft donor area is highly desirable. This allows early re-harvesting of grafts from same donor site which is important in patients with large extent of burns. Effective pain control and avoidance of infection of donor area are other important considerations while planning local management of donor area. Impregnated tulle gras, alginates, collagen sheets are some of the commonly used covers for donor area. A chapter in the section devoted to this topic, describes new approach using banana leaf dressing and polyethylene surgical drape as alternative dressings for donor area. Management of full thickness skin graft donor site with an innovative technique is the topic of the other chapter.

All our authors have extensive experience in this subject. Their insight, involvement and innovative ideas are apparent in their contribution. I sincerely appreciate the commitment of each of the authors and would like to thank all of these experts who have contributed to this book.

I hope the readers would find this book informative and practical. I wish it would provide stimulus to some for development and evaluation of some innovative and imaginative techniques.

Dr. Madhuri Gore
Former Chief of Surgery and Burns,
Lokmanya Tilak Municipal Medical College and General Hospital,
Sion, Mumbai, India.

Section 1

Preparation of Recipient Area

Chapter 1

Hydrosurgery-System® in Burn Surgery – Indications and Applications

Thomas Rappl

Additional information is available at the end of the chapter

http://dx.doi.org/10.5772/51851

1. Introduction

- Apart from the extent and depth of burns, inflammatory reactions and infections (caused by impurities, cell detritus, bacterial degradation etc.) impair the healing of burn wounds. Bacterial colonization and invasion significantly influence wound healing (epithelialisation and contraction of the wound) [1]. Early debridement and depth-specific early coverage are currently the standard in the surgical treatment of burns [2,3,8,10]. Basic prerequisites are exact determination of the depth and accurate debridement. Particularly in cases of large burn wounds it is essential to preserve and protect vital tissue. In cases of wide, generous removal of tissue by the use of the Dermatom, Guilon or Humbey knife, one frequently removes more than the actual burned tissue and unnecessarily damages vital tissue. On the other hand, one may remove too little necrotic tissue. The depth of the burn may be difficult to difficult to assess so that the surgeon waits too long, causing valuable time to lapse during which he may well have performed surgical repair. Accurate ablation of the damaged layers of skin and identification of petechial bleeding help to assess the vitality of tissue. This permits exact determination of depth (whether the subpapillary, cutaneous or subdermal plexus are preserved) [9,16] and depth-specific coverage.
- Versajet® is a hydrosurgical system employing a jet of water by which tissue is simultaneously cut, ablated, and suctioned. The wound is rinsed without significant aerosolisation. This system has been approved by the US Food and Drug Administration (FDA) for debridement of wounds and soft tissue as well as CE-certified for ablation of tissue and other substances in various surgical procedures including wound debridement [7]. The system is based on the Venturi principle: a thin high-velocity jet of water consisting of sterile saline is discharged from a 0.12-mm nozzle into a suction tube (see Table 1). The

consistency of the working tip and the velocity of the water jet create a vacuum below the incision window. This aspirates, cuts and suctions the tissue. As the handpiece is held parallel to the wound the high-pressure water jet acts as a scalpel. When the working tip is tilted slightly the scalpel effect of the water jet is reduced while the rinsing and suction effect is enhanced. Furthermore, the quantity of ablated tissue is determined by the pressure settings at the console (1-10), the pressure exerted by the surgeon, and the speed at which the handpiece is moved on tissue. The console is operated by a foot pedal. Hydrosurgical systems have been in use for a large variety of indications [14]. However, they have not entered burn surgery thus far. Further development of the concept led to a more modern system, namely the Versajet® system, which works precisely and simply. A number of handpieces are currently available for various purposes. They differ in terms of the size of the surgical window and the angle of the working tip: 8 mm surgical window, 45° angle, 14 mm surgical window, 15° or 45° angle of the working tip. Furthermore, the different holders are also available in a Versajet plus® variation which enables the surgeon to forcefully ablate tough tissue.The basic principles underlying this concept were derived from histological investigations. The exact layer-wise removal of tissue components achieved by this procedure is of the same quality as that achieved by laser ablation. The Versajet system® was also successfully used for the treatment and the removal of dirt-tattoos/pigment deposits.

Pressure levels	Flow rate of the jet	Velocity of water pressure
1	90 ml/min	103 bar 426 km/h
3	125 ml/min	265 bar 591 km/h
7	188 ml/min	587 bar 885 km/h
10	230 ml/min	827 bar 1078 km/h

Table 1. Physical data

2. Case 1

Figures 1 to 5 show a 6-year old boy with partial to full thickness scalds in the neck. Large portions of the chest were also affected. Necrosectomy with Versajet® (at levels 5–7) and subsequent coverage with unmeshed split-thickness skin graft were performed on the 4th day after the accident. Fat gauze was placed on the grafts. A collar was provided to protect the grafts and immobilize the neck postoperatively. On the 6th postoperative day the split-thickness skin grafts had healed in a stable manner. Bacterial investigations performed before and after the treatment showed no microbial growth. The functional outcome after six months was favourable.

http://dx.doi.org/10.5772/51851

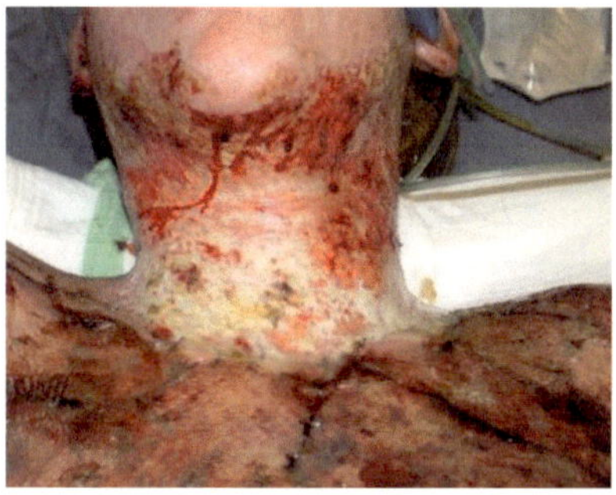

Figure 1. 6-year-old boy, grade partial to full thickness scalds in the chest and neck, 11% of body surface.

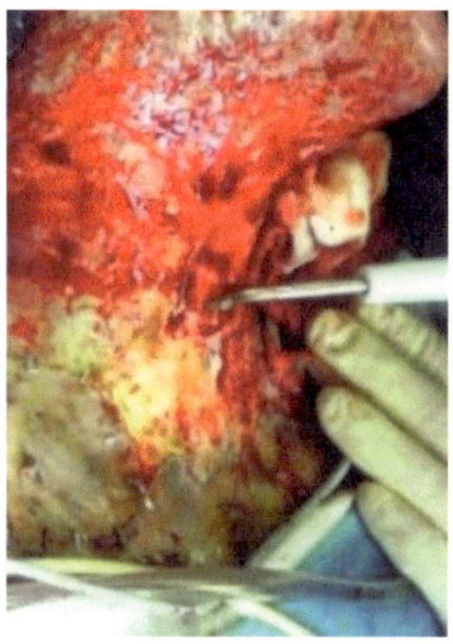

Figure 2. Necrosectomy with Versajet®.

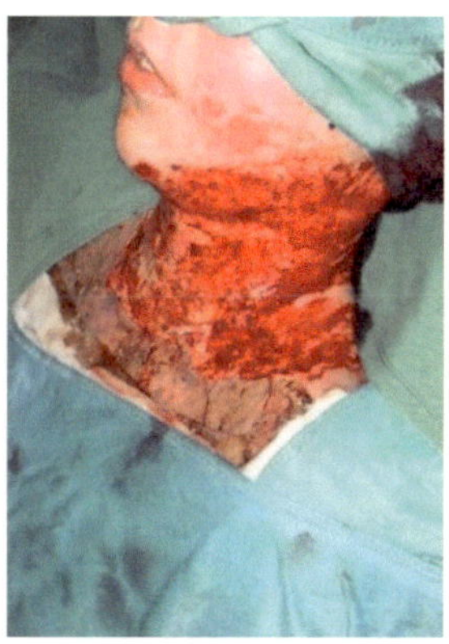

Figure 3. After necrosectomy.

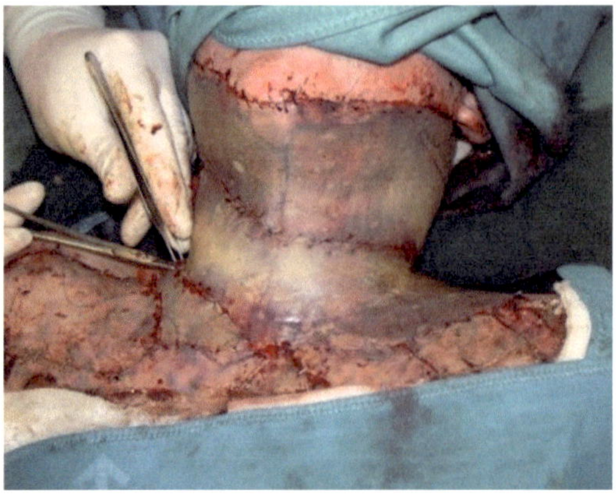

Figure 4. Split-thickness skin graft, unmeshed

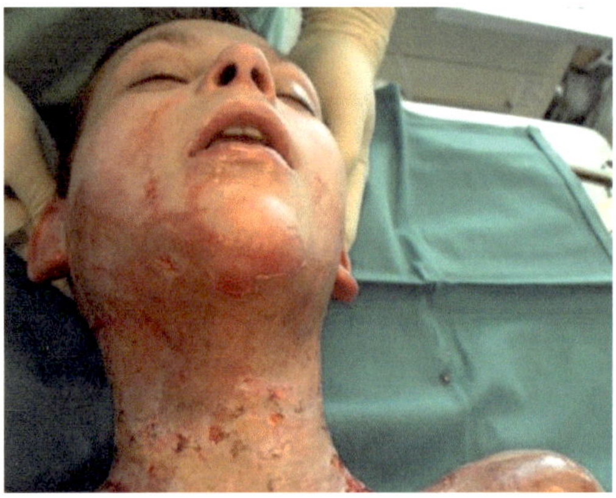

Figure 5. 10 days postoperatively

3. Case 2

Fig. 6 to 10 show a 45-year-old man who developed partial to full thickness-burns in both hands and partial thickness burns in the forearm and face during a car accident. Necrosectomy with Versajet® (at levels 3–5) and split-thickness skin grafting on the dorsum of the left hand were performed on the 2nd day after the accident. The hand covered with a split-thickness skin graft was covered with fat gauze and immobilized with a splint for 6 days. The remaining burned areas were superficially cleaned with Versajet® (at level 3) and treated with Acticoat because the smears showed colonization of germs in the wounds. On the 6th postoperative day the split-thickness skin grafts had healed in a stable manner. The smears showed no microbial growth. Function and aesthetics were satisfactory after six months.

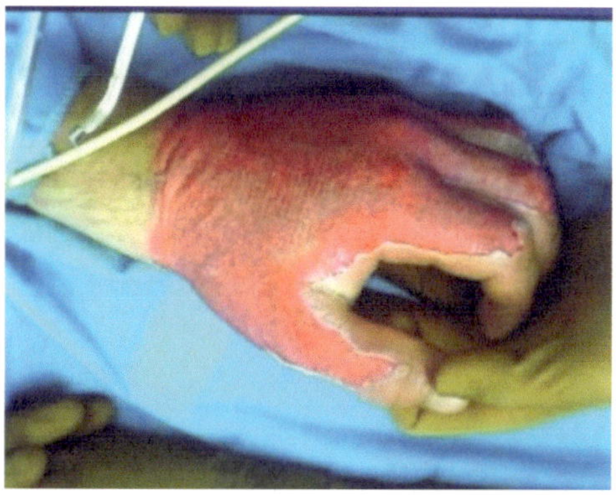

Figure 6. 45-year-old man, grade partial thickness burns on both hands

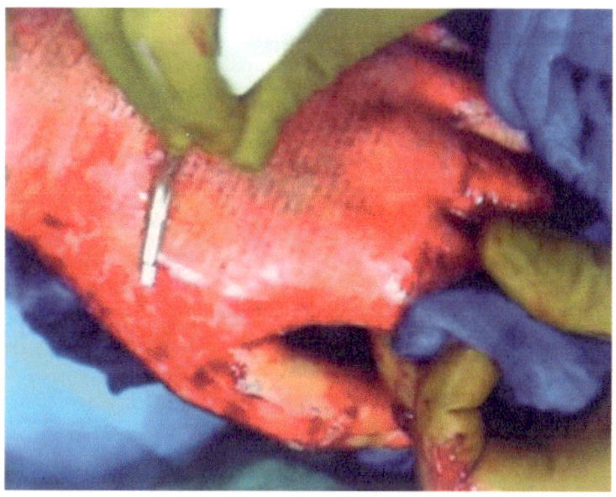

Figure 7. 45-year-old man, grade partial thickness burns on both hands

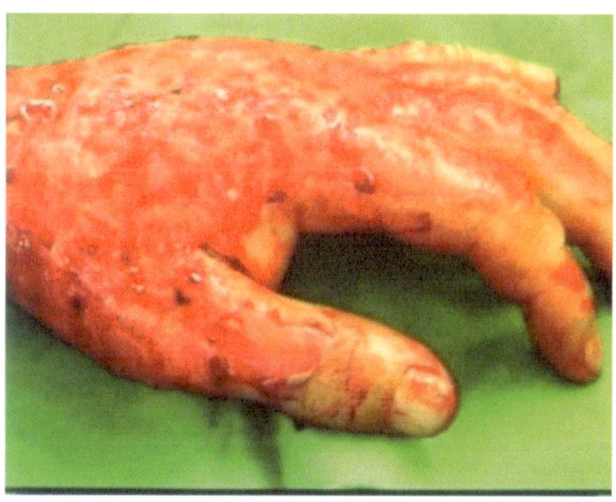

Figure 8. Post debridement

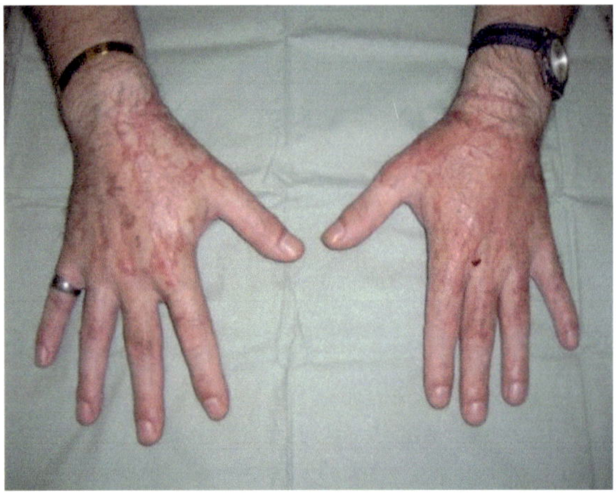

Figure 9. 6 months postoperatively, the left hand is covered with a split-skin graft while the right hand was treated by conservative means

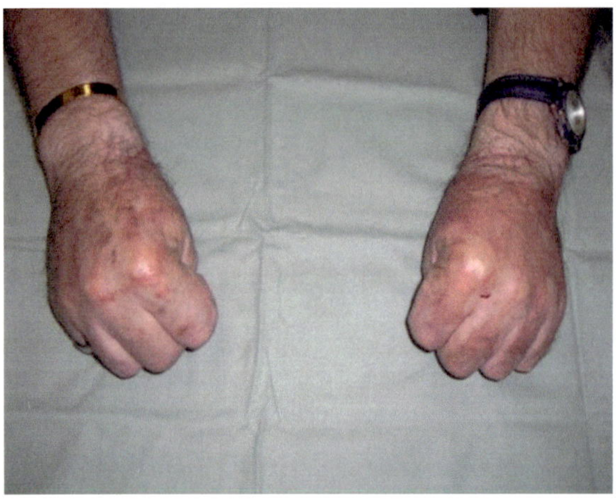

Figure 10. 6 months postoperatively, the left hand is covered with a split-skin graft while the right hand was treated by conservative means

4. Case 3

Fig. 11 to 12 show a 40-year-old man who partial thickness burns in the face covered with pigment deposits after an explosion. Dirt tattoos has been removed by using the hydro surgery system at level 3 with a very superficial removal of the pigment deposits. Uneventful healing shows a clean skin after 2 weeks without scarring.

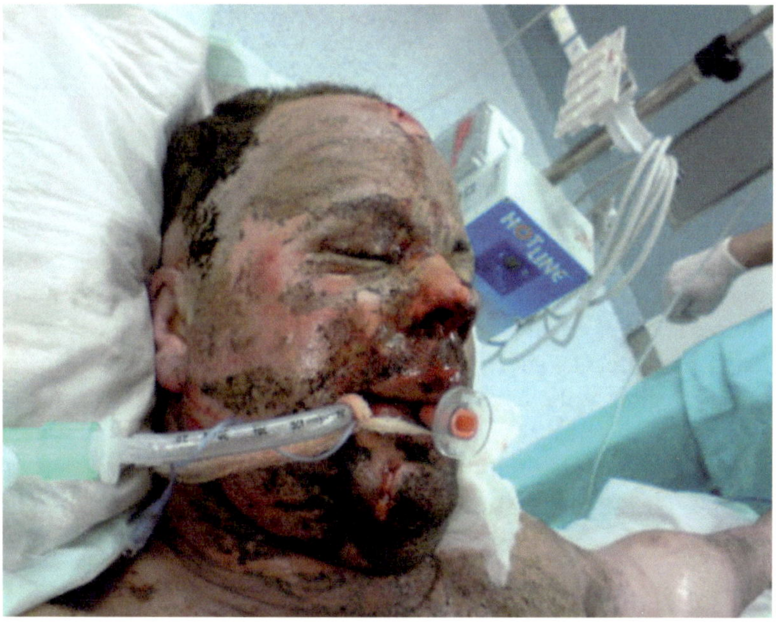

Figure 11.

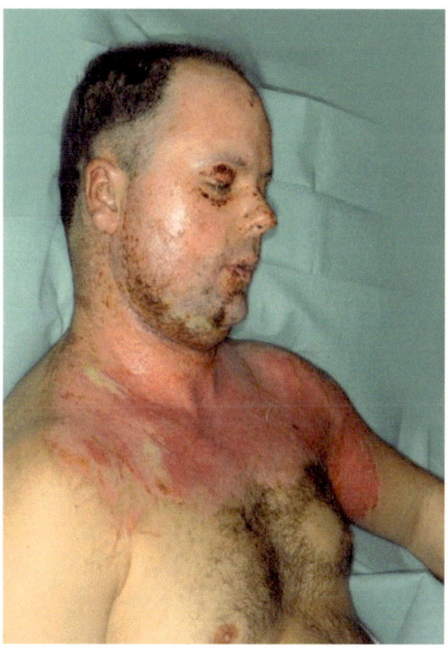

Figure 12.

5. Results

The experience shows that in cases of full thickness burns a necrosectomy with the Dermatom, Humbey knife or the scalpel could be performed rapidly and efficiently. In these cases Versajet® was of use only in marginal zones or to provide the wound with the necessary finishing touches. Tissue damaged in a leathered fashion could not be ablated rapidly or satisfactorily even by the use of Versajet plus®. In contrast, the advantages of Versajet in the treatment of partial thickness burn wounds are worthy of mention. In particular, burns in complex, inaccessible areas are an indication for the use of this hydrosurgical system. In the region of the face (the lips, eyelids, etc.) debridements can be performed with a degree of precision that is hardly achievable by the use of conventional methods. Furthermore, necrosectomy in the region of the hand (fingers, interdigital spaces, etc.) can be significantly improved by the use of Versajet®. In burn surgery convex surfaces could be ablated uniformly and concavities curetted with precision. Pigment deposits could be completely removed. Histological investigations prove and confirm the precision of ablation by the use of Versajet®.

Fig. 13: This technique permits ablation of clearly defined anatomical structures. Removal of the most superficial layers of skin, dermal papillae/papillary dermis (Fig. 13a). Layer of the superficial reticular dermis, removal of the epidermis, the papillary dermis, and superficial portions of the reticular dermis (Fig. 13b). Layer of the mid reticular dermis (Fig. 13c).

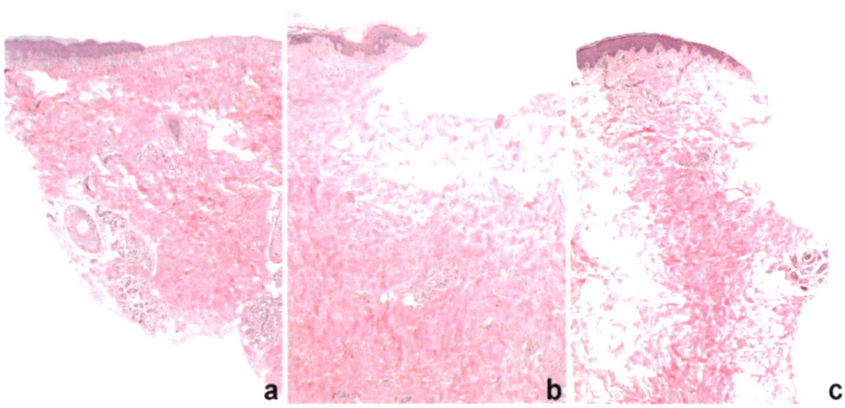

Figure 13. a to c, Layer-wise ablation with Versajet®, a. papillary layer, b reticular layer in the middle, c Reticular layer, deep

In cases of large partial thickness burns this method was very helpful to achieve effective wound debridement. At level 2-3, impurities, coatings and cell detritus could be removed in a simple, rapid and gentle manner and microbial growth could thus be reduced. Smears and

http://dx.doi.org/10.5772/51851

biopsies taken before and after the treatment showed marked reduction of microbial growth in all cases. In superficial wounds that could be treated with Versajet® we observed more rapid re-epithelialisation compared to conservative treatment on the side with the same depth of burns treated with fat gauze. In no case did we encounter side effects or undesired events. Steps, unevenness or ridges in tissue were caused by lack of practice, but could be corrected during the procedure. Postoperative wound dressing was performed according to the general guidelines of burn treatment.

6. Discussion

Surgical debridement as the most common technique for necrosectomy is done using scalpels, forceps, scissors, and other instruments. It is used if your wound is large, has deep tissue damage. It may also be done if debriding the wound is urgent. The skin surrounding the wound is cleaned and disinfected and the damaged tissue is cut away. The wound will be washed out to remove any free tissue. In large damaged areas of full thickness burns, cutting away the entire contaminated wound may be the most rapid and the most effective treatment.

Using *Chemical /enzymatic debridement* a debriding medicine will be applied onto the wound. The wound is then covered with a dressing. The enzymes in the medicine dissolve the dead tissue in the wound. Chemical enzymes are fast acting products that produce slough of necrotic tissue. Some enzymatic debriders are selective, while some are not. Best results are shown on any wound with a large amount of necrotic debris. The main disadvantages of the enzymatic debridement are: costs, a specific secondary dressing may be necessary and sometimes inflammation or discomfort may occur.

Mechanical debridement can involve a variety of methods to remove dead or infected tissue. Allowing a dressing to proceed from moist to wet, then manually removing the dressing causes a form of non-selective debridement. Wet to dry dressing starts by applying a wet dressing to the wound. As this dressing dries, it absorbs wound material. The dressing is then remoistened and removed. Some of the tissue comes with it. This method is useful for wounds with moderate amounts of necrotic debris. This treatment is non-selective and may traumatize healthy or healing tissue, is time consuming and can be painful to patient. Hydrotherapy can cause tissue maceration. Also, waterborne pathogens may cause contamination or infection. Disinfecting additives may be cytotoxic. There are nearly no indications in burn-surgery for this kind of debridement.

Autolytic Debridement uses dressings that retain wound fluids that assist your body's natural abilities to clean the wound. This type of dressing is more often used to treat pressure sores than burns. This process takes more time than other methods. It will not be used for wounds that are infected or if quick treatment is needed. It is a good treatment if the body cannot tolerate more forceful treatments, it's a selective, effective, easy and safe process with no damage to surrounding skin, using the body's own defence mechanisms to clean the wound of necrotic debris, with little to no pain for the patient. But it's not as rapid as surgical debridement, the wound must be monitored closely for signs of infection. Promote anaerobic growth may occur, if an occlusive hydrocolloid is used. Because of the time consuming process we won't recommend this treatment for debridement of burned tissue.

Hydrosurgery permits accurate intraoperative diagnosis of the depth of burns. The petechial bleeding that occurs during necrosectomy shows that the subpapillary plexus is preserved and the burn may be treated by conservative means. Nevertheless, one should not hesitate to perform skin transplantation if necessary because the risk of hypertrophic scar formation is very high when necrosectomy is insufficient and no coverage provided [3]. With regard to superficial wound debridement the hydrosurgical system is superior to other procedures (such as jet lavage) because it simultaneously cleans the wound and carries away the ablated particles without significant aerosolisation. Several methods are available for debridement and conditioning of the wound bed [5, 6]. Sharp physical debridement is of undisputed value for the treatment of full thickness burns. In cases of 28 burns the advantages of Versajet® in respect of handling and precision have been mentioned earlier. Versajet and laser ablation were found to be of equal quality with regard to the depth of layers and accuracy. A major advantage of Versajet® is the duration of the treatment. More than one treatment session is rarely necessary. The achievable outcome is identical on histology as well as gross investigation. In the hands of an experienced user Versajet® has no disadvantages or side effects compared to other methods. In order to achieve the best possible outcome in complex concave or convex regions, a certain amount of experience in using the device is required. Particularly in the eyelids, the surgeon must have sufficient experience in handling the apparatus. The learning curve is quite steep. After a few treatments the operator will be confident enough to treat complex sites at no risk. However, it should be ensured that the settings at the console are initially low (level 3-5) because a higher intensity causes more aggressive ablation, which may be associated with disadvantages such as irregularities and step formation in tissue. In most cases the moderate setting (setting 5-8) is used and has proved to be adequate. As the handpiece is a disposable system, the question of cost-effectiveness arises. However, by using Versajet® early the surgeon is able to rapidly establish the indication for reconstruction. The additional cost is balanced by the fact that the duration of the hospital stay is shortened [7].

7. Conclusion

As rapid debridement and immediate deep coverage should be performed for the reasons mentioned at the beginning of this report as well as to avoid the risk of hypertrophic scar formation [12], Versajet® fulfils standards of precision, rapid intervention and simple handling. The special domain of Versajet® is partial thickness burns, particularly in poorly accessible anatomical regions [4,13]. These regions can be treated and debrided more effectively by the use of hydrosurgical systems than with conventional methods. By means of layer-wise ablation the surgeon is able to identify healthy tissue immediately and protect it in the best possible manner. Intraoperative diagnosis of the depth of burns is also achieved by this procedure. Owing to these advantages the Versajet® system has become a standard procedure in burn surgery.

http://dx.doi.org/10.5772/51851

Author details

Thomas Rappl

Department of Plastic, Aesthetic & Reconstructive Surgery, Medical University Graz, Austria

References

[1] Bojrab MJ: A Handbook on Veterinary Wound Management. Ashland, OH: KenVet Professional Veterinary Company, 1994

[2] Breie Z, Zdrovic F: Lessons learned from 2409 burn patients operated by early excision. Scand J Plast Surg 1979; 13: 107–118

[3] Burke JF, Quimby WC, Bondoc CC: Primary excision and prompt grafting as routine therapy for the treatment of thermal burns in children. Surg Clin N Am 1976; 56: 477–494

[4] Cubison TC, Pape SA, Jeffery SL: Dermal preservation using the Versajet ® hydrosurgery system for debridement of paediatric burns. Burns 2006; 32: 714–720

[5] Eldad A, Weinberg A, Breiterman S, Chaouat M, Palanker D, Ben-Bassat H: Early nonsurgical removal of chemically injured tissue enhances wound healing in partial thickness burns. Burns 1998; 24: 166–172

[6] Falabella AF: Debridement and wound bed preparation. Dermatologic Therapy 2006; 19: 317–325

[7] Granick MS, Possnett JW, Jackoby M, Noruthum S, Ganchi P, Daliashvili R: Efficacy and cost-effectiveness of the high powered parallel water jet for wound debridement. Poster, EWMA, Stuttgart, 2005

[8] Herndon DN, Gore D, Cole M et al.: Determinants of mortality in pediatric patients with greater than 70% full thickness total body surface area thermal injury treated by early total excision and grafting. J Trauma 1987; 27: 208–212

[9] Jackson DM: The diagnosis of the depth of burning. Br J Surg 1953; 40: 588–596

[10] Janzekovic Z: A new concept in the early excision and immediate grafting of burns. J Trauma 1970; 10: 1103–1108

[11] Kamolz LP, Andel H, Haslik W, Winter W, Meissl G, Frey M: Use of subatmospheric pressure therapy to prevent burn wound progression in human: first experiences. Burns 2004; 30: 253–258

[12] McDonald WS, Deitch EA: Hypertrophic skin grafts in burned patients: a prospective analysis of variables. J Trauma 1987; 27: 147–150

[13] Rennekampff H-O, Schaller HE, Wisser D, Tenenhaus M: Debridement of burn wounds with a water jet surgical tool. Burns 2006; 32: 64–69

[14] Shekarriz B, Shekarriz H, Upadhyay J, Wood DP, Bruch HP: Hydro-jet dissection for laparoscopic nephrectomy: a new technique. Urology 1999; 54: 964–967

[15] Sheridan RL, Lydon MM, Petras LM, Schomacker KT, Tompkins RG, Glatter RD, Parrish JA: Laser ablation of burns: initial clinical trial. Surgery 1999; 125: 92–95

[16] Womack BS: Wound management: healing & assessment. Veterinary Technician 2001; 22: 588–594

Section 2

Procedure of Wound Closure With Skin Grafts

Chapter 2

Evaluation of Skin Grafting Procedure in Burnt Patients

Madhuri A. Gore, Meenakshi A. Gadhire and
Sandeep Jain

Additional information is available at the end of the chapter

http://dx.doi.org/10.5772/54184

1. Introduction

Skin grafting is integral to burn wound management and is the only way of providing permanent wound closure of full thickness burn and deep partial thickness burn that fails to heal within 3 weeks. With pre-existing burn wound, paucity of autograft donor site and compromised status of patient, successful autografting is the key to patient survival. With periodic change in the team of surgical trainees working in the burn unit, it was considered necessary to develop a protocol for the skin grafting procedure. Implementation of this protocol was expected to yield uniform outcome despite change in the operating team. Validation of this protocol was considered necessary to evaluate its efficacy. This study was carried out over a period of 22 months from 1st July 2003 to 31st April 2005.

2. Aims & objectives

1. To evaluate the efficacy of the protocol for skin grafting procedure, primary end point being percentage graft take on 8th post grafting day.
2. To assess the difference in efficacy of procedure in relation to time of surgery.
3. To evaluate the need for blood transfusion during the grafting procedure.

3. Materials and methods

The patients with burn injury subjected to Split Skin Grafting over 22 months from 1st July 2003 to 31st April 2005 were studied prospectively. Specially prepared proforma was used for data collection.

The patients were categorized in three groups

Group 1: Early Excision and Grafting: Patients were stabilized and tangential excision of burn wound was done within 2nd to 5th post burn day.

Group 2: Delayed Excision and Grafting: Burn wound was excised and grafted between 10-14 th post burn day.

Group 3: Grafting on Granulating Wounds: Grafting on granulating wound after eschar separation.

The skin grafting procedure was undertaken if the following criteria were satisfied

Afebrile for at least 24 hours

Hemoglobin >8 gm/dl

Serum albumin >2.5gm/dl

No streptococcal growth on wound culture

Procedure Protocol:

- Maximum of 15 to 20 % total body surface area was grafted at one procedure
- Excision of wound or eschar or hypergranulating tissue upto healthy tissue with punctuate bleeding using Humby's knife handle after infiltration of adrenaline:saline 1:300000 solution.
- Hemostasis with saline + adrenaline soaked pads and compression.
- Simultaneous harvesting of split thickness skin grafts from suitable donor site with second Humby's knife and expansion of graft.
- Sprinkling of chloramphenicol powder on recipient area using spoon or salt pepper dispenser. (Fig 1 A and B)
- Application of skin grafts on recipient site.
- Pressing of skin graft with saline soaked gauze.
- Removal of all blood clots from skin grafts on recipient area.
- Covering the grafts with Vaseline and chlorhexidine impregnated tulle grass.
- Cover with single layer of saline soaked gauze.
- Wrapping of gamjee roll.
- Firm bandaging and application of plaster of paris splint for immobilization of part if extremity or neck is involved.
- Donor site dressed with autoclaved banana leaf dressing, gamjee roll and firm bandaging.
- First change of recipient site dressing at 48 hours, variable schedule later. Donor site dressing change on 8th post op day.

The data was analyzed at the end of study period.

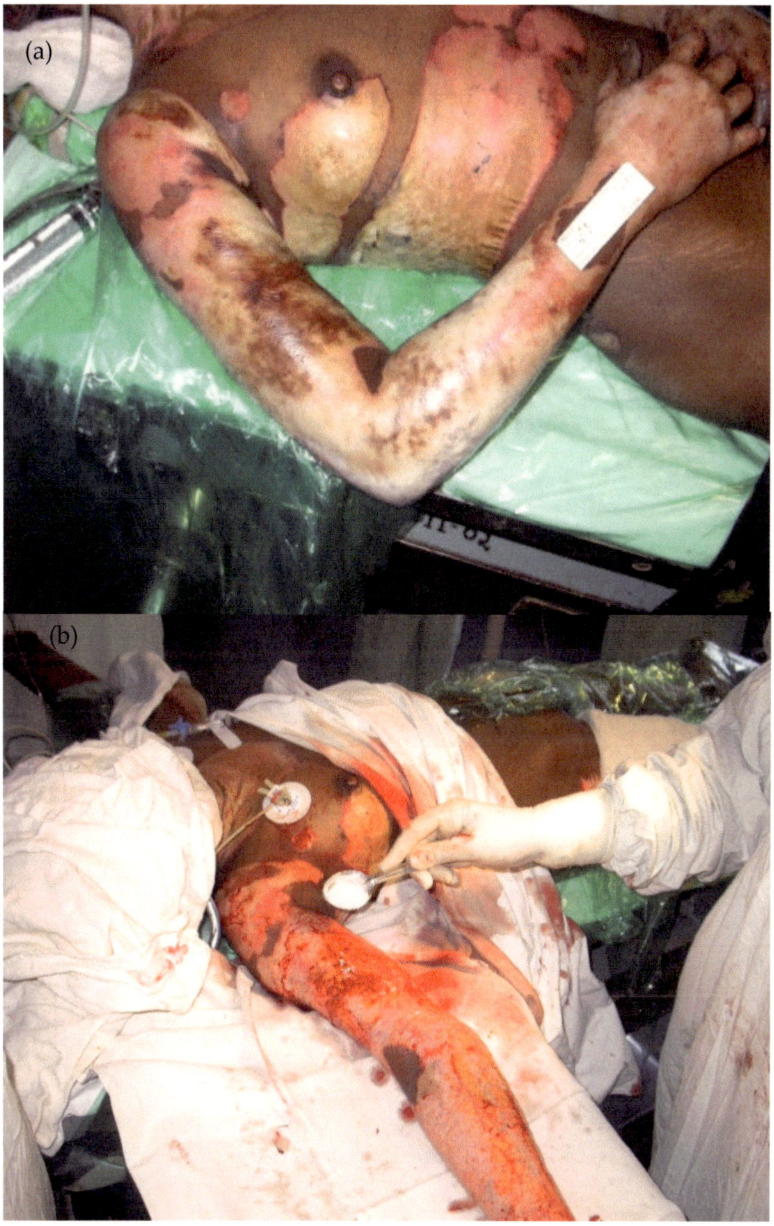

Figure 1. Showing Wound bed preparation. A : Burn wound before early excision; B: Sprinkling of Chloramphenicol powder after adequate excision of burn wound

4. Results

This study included 214 patients subjected to skin grafting procedure. Majority of the patients were adult females (76.2%). Adult males were 15.9% while children comprised 7.9% of the patients. The ratio of females : males : children was 9.6 : 2: 1. Total extent of burn ranged from 5-70% TBSA. (Table 1)

Patient group	No. of patients (%)	Burn size range/ Average extent %TBSA	No. of procedures
Pediatric(male+ female)	17 (7.9%)	5-28% (13%)	17 (6.7%)
Adult male	34 (15.9%)	6-70% (28%)	42 (16.5%)
Adult female	163 (76.2%)	10-70% (40%)	196 (76.8%)
Total	214		255

TBSA – Total Body Surface Area

Table 1. Showing distribution of patients, burn extent and procedures

A total of 255 skin grafting procedures were performed in these 214 patients divided in three groups; early excision and grafting, delayed excision and grafting, grafting on granulating wounds. (Table 2)

Type of procedure	Number of procedures	Number of patients
Early excision & grafting	14 (5.5%)	11 (5.1%)
Delayed excision & grafting	142 (55.7%)	106 (49.5%)
Grafting on granulating wound	99 (38.8%)	97 (45.3%)
Total	255	214

Table 2. Showing distribution of patients and procedures

Deep partial thickness and full thickness burn wounds ranging from 4-30% TBSA were grafted during either a single or more number of procedures.

Early Excision and Grafting: 14 procedures were done in 11 patients with the first procedure within 72 hours of burn injury. 3 patients required the procedure twice due to the extent of burn wound.

Delayed Excision and Grafting: 142 procedures were done in 106 patients more than 10 days after receiving the burn injury. Single procedure was done in 70 patients. 36 patients required the procedure twice due to either partial graft rejection or extensive total burn surface area. In this group 2 patients expired due to systemic sepsis.

http://dx.doi.org/10.5772/54184

Grafting of Granulating Wounds: Granulating wounds of 97 patients required 99 procedures of skin grafting more than 3 weeks after the burn injury. 2 patients required the procedure twice. (Table: 3)

Average graft take in this series was 85% and average requirement of blood transfusion was 2.1 units per procedure.

Donor area infection was found in only 1 patient in delayed excision and grafting group. Duration of donor area epithelization was 9-12 days with an average of 10 days

5. Discussion

In this study, 255 skin grafting procedures performed on 214 burnt patients were analysed and evaluated. Majority of the patients were females (76.2%) with average burn extent (40% TBSA) larger than males (28% TBSA) (Table 1) This has been the consistent observation at our burn unit.

Skin grafting is an integral part of burn wound management and is the only way of providing permanent skin closure for full thickness and deep partial thickness burn wounds. Closure of burn wound has been described at various stages of healing- early excision & grafting, delayed excision & grafting and grafting on granulating wounds after spontaneous separation of eschar.

'Early closure' of burn wounds by excising the burned tissues and promptly covering it with skin-grafts or its substitutes within first 'five' post-burns day is the standard of care today.[1,2] and should ideally be offered to all minor burns and for the major burns who are admitted to a well-equipped burns centre.[3] In addition to improvement in the prognosis, early excision and grafting procedures have been shown to decrease the duration of hospitalization, incidence of metabolic complications, blood transfusion requirements, burn wound contamination, post burn contractures and cost of burn treatment.[4,5,6,7] But large number of patients with large extent of burn and paucity of trained surgeons are the chief factors that make it difficult for us to perform early excisions routinely at our burn unit. In the present study only 11 (5.1%) patients were subjected to early excision and grafting contributing to 14 (5.5%) procedures out of 255.(Table 2)

Burn-wound excision and closure beyond 6 days to 11th or 12th day post-burn still offers "primary intention healing" of the burn-wounds.[2] Our experience indicates that delayed excision & grafting is a feasible and suitable option for patients at our unit with the constraints that we face. We prefer to do it 10 th postburn day onwards. This allows healing of most of the superficial partial thickness burns, thus effectively reducing the total extent of burn. The eschar is well formed and hence is technically easier to excise (Fig 2 A and B). In this series majority of patients i.e. 106(49.5%) were subjected to 142 (55.7%) delayed excision and skin grafting procedures.

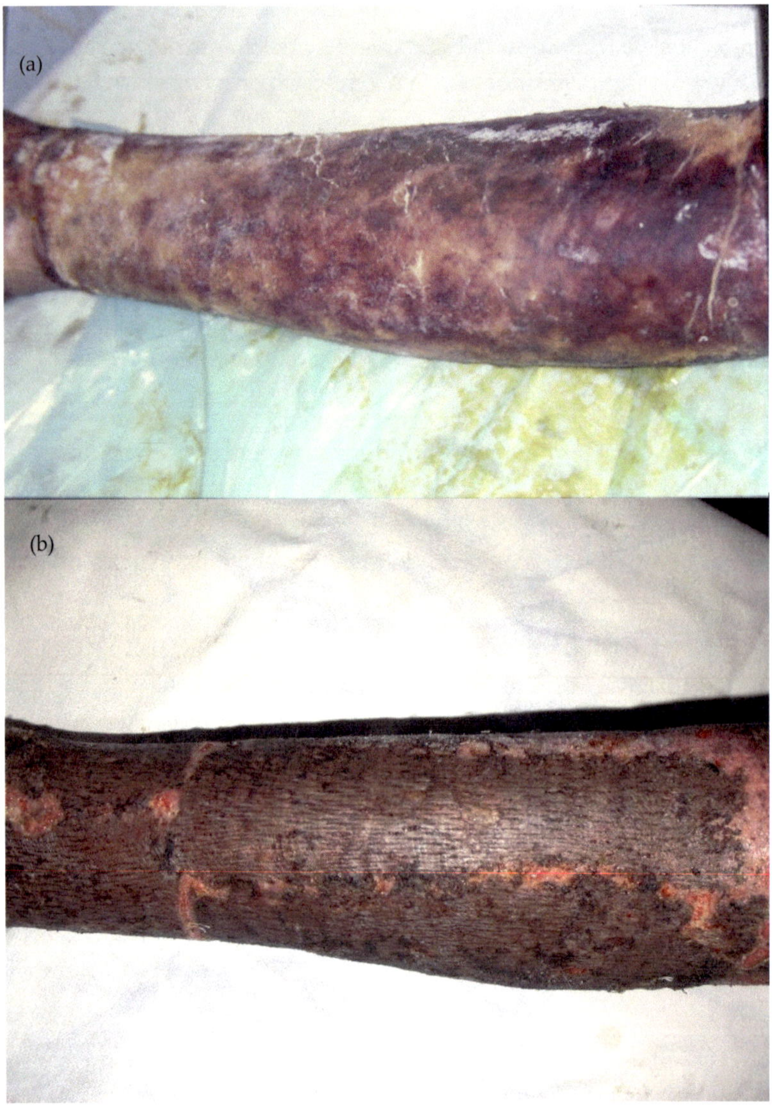

Figure 2. Delayed excision and skin grafting. A: Dry eschar on full thickness burn wound before excision; B: Graft take on 8 th day after excision and grafting

The patients who were unsuitable for both of the above options most often due to infectious complications, were the candidates for grafting after spontaneous separation of eschar and granulation of wound. In this group 99(38.8%) procedures were performed in 97 (45.3%) patients. (Table 2)

The surgical trainees are posted in the burns unit by rotation. With this changing team, having a defined protocol for skin grafting procedure was considered appropriate.

The chief thought was to keep the protocol simple and cheap.

We decided to accept Haemoglobin level of 8 gm% or more for conducting the procedure and found no reason to regret the decision. Agarwal et al [8] have reported similar observations.

All patients were receiving enteral nutritional supplement and we accepted serum albumin level of 2.5 gms% or more. Mogazy et al have reported better correlation between serum pre-albumin levels and graft take in burnt patients[9]. But we have no experience about this.

Several methods like use of fibrin glue to negative pressure device have been described for fixing the graft to the wound bed. In the experience of the first author, Choramphenicol powder acts like a glue as it becomes sticky on contact with recipient site. This helps in fixation of the grafts without use of sutures or staples and helps cut the time and the cost of the procedure without compromising the graft take. Immobilization of the patient in the bed is ensured for atleast first 48 hours post grafting.

Vaseline and Chlorhexidine impregnated tulle gras –readily available in the institution was used as the first layer to cover the skin grafts according to the protocol. Though the literature describes use of Xeroform[10], Acticoat[11], these materials are expensive and difficult to procure for our patient population. No reports of controlled trials are available for comparison.

One of the key factors for the success of skin grafting procedure is removal of dead tissue and adequate preparation of recipient area. The adequacy of excision and harvesting of skin grafts was demonstrated, assisted and/or supervised by the senior surgeons in the team for each procedure.

The average take of skin graft was 95% (range 85-100%) in early excision and grafting group. It was 85% (range 60-90%) in delayed excision and grafting group and was 90% (range 65-100%) when grafting of granulating wounds was performed.(Table3) The average graft take was 85% in all the procedures performed. Literature search did not reveal much information to compare our observations. But with average 85% graft take, our protocol for skin grafting procedure can be considered effective.

The requirement for transfusion of packed red blood cells during surgery or within 2 days post-procedure was the lowest (1.2 unit, range 0-3 units) in early excision and grafting group. It was the highest (2.9 units, range 0-5 units) when granulating wounds were grafted and the delayed excision and grafting group required average 2.4 units (range 1-4 units). (Table 3)

	Early Excision & Grafting	Delayed Excision & Grafting	Grafting of Granulating Wound
No. of procedures	14	142	99
No. of patients	11	106	97
Grafted burn size	4-23% TBSA	7-30% TBSA	3-17% TBSA
Transfusion requirement in units/ procedure (average in units)	0-3 (1.1)	1-4 (2.4)	0-5 (2.9)
Graft take % (average %)	85-100 (95%)	60-90 (85%)	65-100 (90%)

TBSA : Total Body Surface Area

Table 3. Showing procedures, graft take and transfusion requirement

Two patients in the delayed excision and grafting group died within 8 days of the procedure due to multi-organ failure due to systemic sepsis.

The donor area healing was satisfactory under banana leaf dressing. This dressing has been developed and evaluated at the burn unit earlier[12].

6. Conclusions

The results of our study suggest that

1. Our protocol for skin grafting procedure is effective with average graft take of 85% with application of the protocol.
2. Early excision and skin grafting was the most successful procedure with 95% graft take.
3. Early excision and skin grafting group had the least transfusion requirement amongst the three groups.

Author details

Madhuri A. Gore*, Meenakshi A. Gadhire and Sandeep Jain

*Address all correspondence to: drmadhuri@hotmail.com

Burn Care Service, Department of Surgery, LTM Medical College and Hospital, Sion, Mumbai, India

References

[1] A retrospective analysis of early excision and skin grafting from 1993-1995.Chamania S, Patidar GP, Dembani B, Baxi M. Burns. 1998 Mar;24(2):177-80.

[2] Delayed primary closure of the burn wounds. Prasanna M, Mishra P, Thomas C. Burns. 2004 Mar;30(2):169-75

[3] Early tangential excision and skin grafting as a routine method of burn wound management: an experience from a developing country. Prasanna M, Singh K, Kumar P Burns. 1994 Oct;20(5):446-50.

[4] Rationale for early tangential excision and grafting in burn patients. Kisslaogglu E, Yuksel F, Uccar C, Karacaogglu E. Acta Chir Plast. 1997;39(1):9-12.

[5] Early excision of major burns in children: effect on morbidity and mortality. Pietsch JB, Netscher DT, Nagaraj HS, Groff DB. J Pediatr Surg. 1985 Dec;20(6):754-7

[6] Early burn excision and grafting. Heimbach DM. Surg Clin North Am. 1987 Feb; 67(1):93-107

[7] Primary excision of the burn wound. Still JM Jr, Law EJ Clin Plast Surg. 2000 Jan; 27(1):23-47, v-vi .

[8] Evaluation of skin graft take following post-burn raw area in normovolaemic anaemia, Pawan Agarwal, Brijesh Prajapati, and D. Sharma; Indian J Plast Surg. 2009 Jul-Dec; 42(2): 195–198.

[9] Assessment of the relation between prealbumin serum level and healing of skin-grafted burn wounds. Moghazy AM, Adly OA, Abbas AH, Moati TA, Ali OS, Mohamed BA. Burns. 2010 Jun;36(4):495-500.

[10] Management of skin-grafted burn wounds with Xeroform and layers of dry coarse-mesh gauze dressing results in excellent graft take and minimal nursing time. Hansbrough W, Doré C, Hansbrough JF. J Burn Care Rehabil. 1995 Sep-Oct;16(5):531-4.

[11] A silver-coated antimicrobial barrier dressing used postoperatively on meshed autografts: a dressing comparison study. Silver GM, Robertson SW, Halerz MM, Conrad P, Supple KG, Gamelli RL. J Burn Care Res. 2007 Sep-Oct;28(5):715-9.

[12] Banana Leaf dressing for skin graft donor areas; Gore M A; Akolekar D; Burns 2003 (29): 483 – 486

Chapter 3

The Fixation and Dressing for Meshed and Sheet Skin Graft

Yoshiaki Sakamoto and Kazuo Kishi

Additional information is available at the end of the chapter

http://dx.doi.org/10.5772/52472

1. Introduction

When a graft is placed on a recipient bed, the process of accepting the graft begins. For some hours, the graft is bathed and nourished by plasmatic circulation or serum imbibition. Simultaneously, fortuitous and accidental apposition of the vessels in the bed and those in the graft allows blood to be sucked into the graft. Soon afterwards, active penetration of the graft by blood vessels from the bed begins and is well-established by the fifth day. These 5 days are the most important period for skin graft acceptance.

In other words, to improve the survival of the transplanted skin graft, it is important to ensure that the graft is not misaligned with the recipient bed and that moderate pressure is applied on the transplanted skin so that it is in contact with and adheres to the recipient bed. These measures are achieved through fixation and dressing. This chapter will cover various types of fixations and dressings.

2. Fixation of skin grafts

With the exception of particular skin grafting methods, such as those used in skin chip grafts, fixation is essential to prevent the skin graft from being misaligned with the recipient bed, whether the graft is a mesh skin graft or a sheet skin graft. The following sections enumerate 3 such methods and describe their respective advantages and disadvantages. Of course, these methods can also be used in combination with each other.

2.1. Suturing

The most cost-effective and common method is to fix the skin grafts with unabsorbable sutures (Figure 1). This is the most basic method, but its disadvantage are that it is very time consuming because the sutures are sewn one by one and that the removal of the stitches is time-consuming. In addition, if there is epithelialization of the anchoring suture in a mesh skin graft, the suture will be buried in the skin and will be difficult to remove. On rare occasions, because of the thinness of the skin, the sutures may cause stitch abscesses if they are left in place. Therefore, methods involving absorbable sutures are used in order to avoid these issues (Figure 2). In such cases, there is no need to remove the sutures, and no problem occurs even if the anchoring site is epithelialized. However, the suturing time remains the same. Therefore, fixation with an unabsorbable suture is useful in the case of sheet skin grafts, whereas fixation with an absorbable suture is useful in the case of mesh skin grafts.

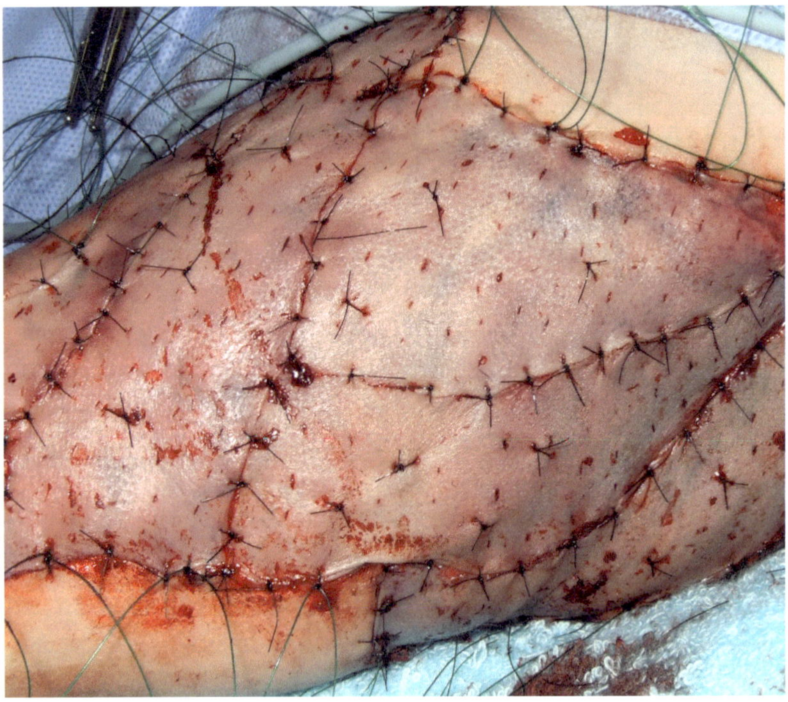

Figure 1. Graft fixation with nylon

http://dx.doi.org/10.5772/52472

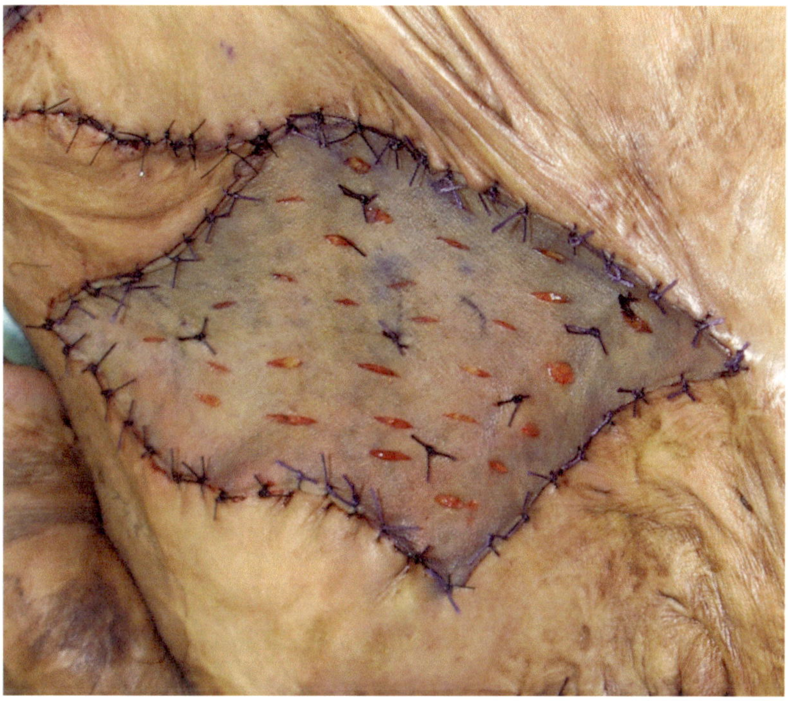

Figure 2. Graft fixation with absorbable sutures.

2.2. Surgical stapler

The greatest advantage of this method is that it is not time-consuming. For this reason, it is used for various purposes, such as when the skin graft extends over a wide area or when the surgeon wants to complete the surgery as early as possible because of the patient's overall condition (Figure 3). However, there are 2 disadvantages: patients often complain of pain during the removal of the sutures and if a mesh skin graft is used in the same way as in the case of fixation using the aforementioned unabsorbable sutures and if epithelialization extends to the stapled sites, then the removal of the sutures will become very difficult.

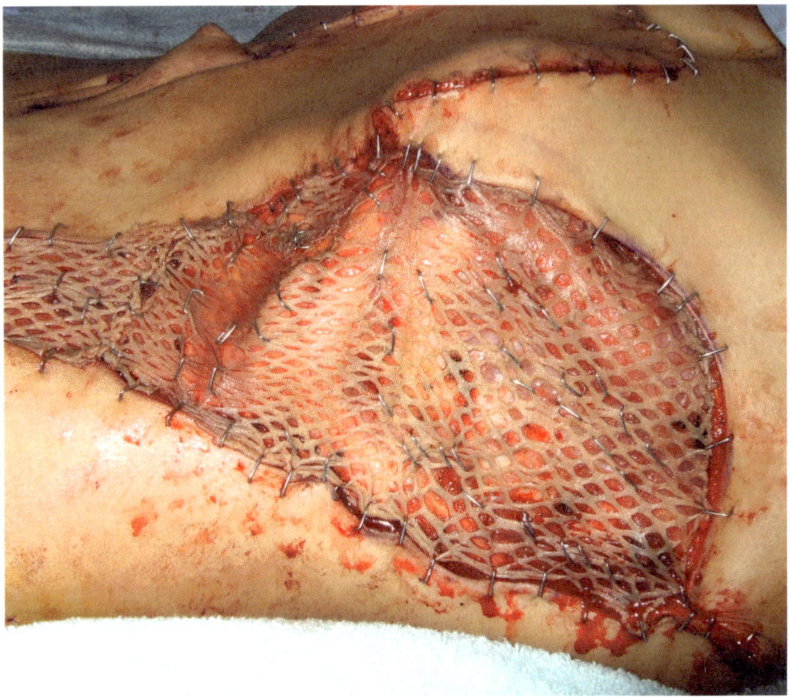

Figure 3. Graft Fixation with skin stapler

2.3. Octyl-2-cyanoacrylate

This is a new fixation method that we have devised, and it consists of fixing the skin graft by using octyl-2-cyanoacrylate at the time of closing of the surgical wound (Figure 4). As in the case of the staplers, this procedure can be performed in a short time and there is no need for suture removal; therefore, this method is suitable for children. The disadvantage of this method is that it is expensive.

3. Dressing of skin grafts

The dressing of a skin graft has more influence on graft survival than on graft fixation. The main purpose of dressing is to ensure circumferential contact between the graft and the host bed. Ideally, all skin grafts should be accepted; however, complications such as hematoma, movement, and infection occur, notwithstanding the pressure on the skin graft. In addition, pressure necrosis can occur if too much pressure is applied to give priority to adhesion. And a pressure of 30 mmHg was optimal for graft take because it totally compressed venous vascularization and partially compressed arterial vascularization [1).

In the following section, various dressing methods have been discussed; however, regardless of the method used, the dressing is usually left in place for approximately 5 days. If the transplanted skin and the dressing adhere to each other at the time of change of the first dressing, the transplanted skin that has adhered to the recipient bed could end up getting peeled off. Therefore, a non-adherent siliconized gauze is placed directly onto the transplanted skin to prevent it from adhering to the dressing.

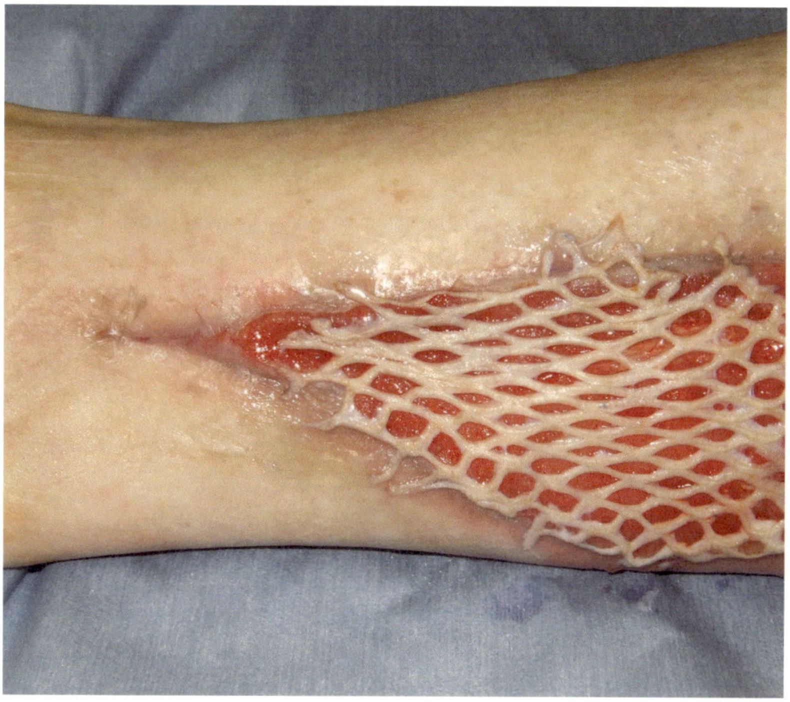

Figure 4. Graft fixation with Octyl-2-cyanoacrylate

3.1. Simple pressure dressing

This is the most basic skin graft fixation method. It is indicated for flat and poorly operational areas. This method consists of placing a silicon gauze on the skin graft and laying a piece of cotton or gauze on top to compress the skin graft. Fixation is ensured by compression with tapes or bandages.

3.2. Tie over dressing

A tie-over dressing is the most optimal and reliable technique. In the past, tie-over fixation seemed to be the standard procedure for skin grafting; however, comparison with simple pressure dressing has been reported to show no difference in terms of graft survival [2]. Therefore, this method is basically indicated for locations where tapes are difficult to attach, including mobile areas such as the shoulders, concave and convex surfaces such as the face, and the scalp. The method is performed as follows. Traditionally, nylon sutures are applied along the borders of the graft. The threads of the sutures are long. Next, the graft is dressed with nonadherent gauze, and a bolus of cotton is placed over the graft. Then, the threads on the opposite side are tied together and secured in order to establish a pressure dressing. Regarding cotton, 2 options are available: nylon cotton and raw cotton. If raw cotton is used, moderate pressure can easily be achieved by spreading a wetted piece of raw cotton directly onto non-adherent gauze and by placing fluffy and raw cotton on top. However, because the exudate will be absorbed by the cotton, odor could be an issue and there is risk of infection. However, if nylon cotton is used, there is less risk of infection because the exudate soaks the gauze located on the nylon cotton, which cannot be contaminated because of the capillary phenomenon. Meanwhile, a certain extent of skills is required for the fastening.

The disadvantages of the conventional technique are that the long sutures require time and effort for securing the suture ends. Furthermore, once a conventional tie-over dressing is removed, another similar tie-over dressing cannot be placed on the graft. Furthermore, the stitch marks surrounding the skin graft are unfortunately a common problem. Several unique suturing techniques have been reported as a solution for these issues; but the method described below is the best strategy.

3.3. Negative-pressure dressing

In terms of wound healing, negative-pressure wound closure has been the focus of attention. Since this dressing method uses the principle of negative pressure, we have named it "negative-pressure dressing" (NPD). The greatest advantages of NPD are that it is not time-consuming and that it can be used at locations where tie-over and simple pressure fixation are difficult to achieve as well as in areas with a complex morphology. It can be performed regardless of the size of the skin graft. And it is said the rates of graft loss may be lower when NPD is used [3].

For the procedure, preparations are performed in accordance with the conventional NPWC, and for pressure, a sponge and a film are used. As stated above, this method also requires the use of silicon gauze, which must be sandwiched between the sponge and the skin graft. And the sponge have to be cut its size same as the defect area. Then the sponse is put on the middle of the film, and the sponse and film push over the graft. So you can avoid the movement of graft over recipient site during application of sponge and film over it.

Basically, negative pressure of about 25 to 75 mmHg is applied for 5 consecutive days. Management is easy because, during that time, there is no need to replace the dressing. Even in the case of skin grafting at an infectious site at which the condition of the skin graft needs to be checked once every 2 or 3 days, dressing with NPD can be removed d and then be applied again. At that time, a sponge and suction disk change to new ones. However, if NPD is used continuously over a period of 1 week or longer in order to give priority to the survival of the skin graft, an ulcer may develop.

The use of NPD is contraindicated on the scalp, where it is difficult for the film to adhere, and on the penis and the fingers and toes, where problems with blood flow may develop. In addition, NPD is not used for the fixation of very small-sized skin grafts because of cost issues.

http://dx.doi.org/10.5772/52472

4. Conclusion

In the above chapter, fixation and dressing of skin grafts were discussed. Although these are the most basic methods, they are extremely important and can influence the survival of skin grafts. In addition, various ideas to improve the survival rate of skin grafts have been reported. We hope that our readers will also report new methods in the future.

Author details

Yoshiaki Sakamoto* and Kazuo Kishi

*Address all correspondence to: ysakamoto@z8.keio.jp

Department of Plastic and Reconstructive Surgery, Keio University School of Medicine, Tokyo, Japan

References

[1] Smith, F. A rational management of skin grafts. Surg Gynecol Obstet (1926).

[2] Pulvermacker, B, Chaouat, M, Seroussi, D, & Mimoun, M. Tie-over dressings in full-thickness skin grafts. Dermatol Surg. (2008). , 34, 40-43.

[3] Webster, J, Scuffham, P, Sherriff, K. L, Stankiewicz, M, & Chaboyer, W. P. Negative pressure wound therapy for skin grafts and surgical wounds healing by primary intention. Cochrane Database Syst Rev. (2012). CD009261.

Chapter 4

One Stage Allogenic Acellular Dermal Matrices (ADM) and Split-Thickness Skin Graft with Negative Pressure Wound Therapy

Hyunsuk Suh and Joon Pio Hong

Additional information is available at the end of the chapter

http://dx.doi.org/10.5772/53304

1. Introduction

After first success of epidermal autotransplantation onto a granulating wound in 1869, skin graft become a standard option for closing defect that cannot be closed primarily. [1] Skin graft can be used in various clinical situations. For the reconstruction of traumatic wounds, burn wound, soft tissue defect or skin defect after cancer ablation surgery or after removal of pigmented skin lesion, diabetic wounds and after scar contracture release and pigmented scar removal, skin graft are widely used around the world.

1.1. Skin graft types

1.1.1. Split-thickness skin graft or full-thickness skin grafts

Skin grafts are generally classified as either split-thickness or full-thickness grafts. Split-thickness skin graft includes varying amounts of dermis whereas a full-thickness graft includes the entire dermis. The amount of dermis within the graft determines the likelihood of survival and the degree of contracture. Split-thickness grafts can survive in conditions with less vascularity, but they have a greater likelihood of contracture. In contrast, full-thickness grafts require a better vascular bed for survival but undergo less contracture. Contracture involves contraction of a healed graft and is caused by myofibroblast activity. The thinner the skin graft is, the greater the contracture of the graft. Granulating wounds or skin defect left to heal secondarily, without any grafting, will eventually demonstrate the greatest degree of contracture and are most prone to hypertrophic scarring. [2] The success of skin graft depends on the ability of the grafted skin to receive nutrients in first few days and, subsequently, vascular ingrowth from the recipient bed. Because the full-thickness skin graft is thicker, survival of the graft demands more well-vascularized bed.

The ultimate goal of skin grafting is first to achieve aesthetic results similar to the adjacent recipient site in terms of color, texture and thickness of skin with minimal contractures. Second is to achieve complete "take" of graft, which is closely related to minimal scar tissue formation. The third goal is to make minimal scar on the donor site. [3]

The full-thickness skin graft has superior result than split-thickness skin graft in aesthetic aspects. It has minimal contractures. We can achieve best esthetic results by doing the full-thickness skin graft for all kinds of full-thickness skin defects if there is unlimited donor sites and complete graft "take". But donor site for the full-thickness skin harvest is limited. The size of full-thickness skin is also limited. Even if there is unlimited supply of full-thickness skins, we cannot use it for all kinds of recipient beds because full-thickness graft demands more perfusion from the recipient bed. For these reasons, split-thickness skin grafts are commonly used for most of large skin defects. But the major disadvantage to traditional split-thickness skin graft is related to donor site morbidity, including permanent scar formation. Unfortunately, the thicker the harvested split-thickness skin, the more donor site morbidity that results. These issues are compounded in those with thin skin such as the young patients and in those with limited donor sites that will require serial reharvesting of each donor site after epithelialization. In cases in which grafted sites are frequently exposed, one may consider the aesthetic limitations of a split-thickness skin graft to be less favorable compared with thicker graft.

2. Allogenic dermis with skin graft

To mimic a full-thickness graft and to minimize donor site morbidity, the addition of an allogenic acellular dermal matrix (ADM) to the split-thickness graft can be considered. The use of STSG combined with a layer of allogenic ADM underneath provides an additional layer of tissue coverage and the potential benefit of promoting the imbibition phase of wound healing.

A vascular linkage to allogenic AMD is achieved within 3 days after transplantation as compared with 2 to 3 weeks observed in alternative materials that are manufactured from animal skin. Accordingly, in cases in which the autograft segment was transplanted simultaneously, biointegration is achieved with a vascular linkage on the third day. [4] allogenic ADM has been used in a wide range of areas including soft tissue extensions for cosmetic purposes, skin grafts for patients with burns and replacement of tympanic membrane, nasal septum, and dura mater. Recent studies have shown that application of allogenic ADM is cosmetically and functionally excellent compared with conventional split thickness skin graft. This is because it is effective in maintaining texture and elasticity of the skin tissue by enhancing the underlying dermis. [5-7] When used as a graft, it is repopulated and revascularized by the recipient's cells and supports the survival of an overlying split-thickness skin graft. [5]

3. Why allogenic dermis?

Many acellular dermal substitutes are used clinically. The 3D matrices should enable progressive vascularization and fibroblast invasion from the surrounding tissues. Bovine collagen and porcine collagen are used especially in wound treatment and skin reconstruction. Nevertheless, porcine collagen is regaining interest, with as big advantage the absence of Prion diseases, the porcine viruses also needed to be considered, and porcine collagen might elicit more foreign body reactions than bovine collagen. The animal acellular dermal matrix is commercialized as MatriDerm consists of collagen (bovine dermis) coated with elastin hydrolysate from the ligamentum nuchae. But MatriDerm seems to degrade sooner after 3 months, and no statistical evidence of long-term clinical effectiveness after 1 year. [8,9]

Histological analysis of the underlying allograft derrnal matrix after composite allodermis and skin graft revealed that there were infiltration of host fibroblasts and neovascularization into the allodermis in the absence of an inflammatory cell infiltrate. There were minimal histological differences noted between the allodermis and the dermal component of the control skin graft. Electron-microscopic analysis on day 16 postgraft demonstrates the presence of an intact basement membrane at the junction of the allograft derrnal matrix, similar to that seen on the dermal component of the control site STSG. Keratinocytes had migrated across and attached to the basement membrane, as shown by the presence of hemidesmosomes. Collagen fibers showed typical ultrastructural characteristics, as defined by fiber diameter, banding and orientation. Most importantly, the processed dermal matrix remains and supports the infiltration of host fibroblasts with typical morphological characteristics of normal synthetic fibroblasts. [5]

These findings suggest that the supplemental dermis supplied by the allogenic acellular dermal matrix, which remains and works as matrix, can potentially improve the healing characteristics of an autograft. The clinically relevant implication is the potential for closure of an extensively burned patient using minimal autograft skin, but resulting in a skin cover whose quality is superior to that typically obtained with thin autografts with their tendency for scarring and contracture.

3.1. Human donor skins for dermal grafting

Human acellular dermal matrices (ADM) are derived from human dermis, treated to remove all immunogenic elements: keratinocytes, fibroblasts, vascular endothelium, and smooth muscle cells. Virus screening is also obliged. However, several different technical methods for processing those matrix have been developed, [10,11,12] all aiming to preserve the integrity of the remaining dermal elements as good as possible. The main elements of all ADM are the collagen and elastin fibers, which serve as a 3D natural matrix for the invasion of the native cellular elements in vivo. The amount of remaining growth factors, cytokines depends on the processing method. The first ADM were processed by trypsin, [10,13] freeze-thawing, [11,12] or long incubations with enzymes. Most of those matrix remained highly antigenic, which lead to poor graft survival. [10,11,12,13,14,15] Several different products are currently available for wound care.

1. AlloDerm® (Lifecell Corp., Branchburg, NJ) is an acellular de-epidermalized dermis product that is a semipermanent skin substitute. It is a cryopreserved and lyophilized allodermis that acts strictly as a dermal replacement. It has no protective epidermal analogue. AlloDerm® does become incorporated into the host by tissue ingrowth. AlloDerm® is a freeze-dried cryopreserved acellular dermal matrix on an intact basement membrane complex obtained by processing human donor skin in a saline solution (sodium dodecyl sulfate) and enzymes. [5,15-19] It is decellularized, freeze-dried, and biochemically stabilized, and has been successful alone and in combination with cultured autografts (two-steps procedure) in the treatment of burn wounds and dermal defects. Additionally, AlloDerm® is procured by cryopreservation which may affect the integrity of the elastin matrix, and its manufacturing is expensive.

2. DermaMatrix™ (Synthes, Inc., West Chester, PA) [20,21] is human donor skin processed using a combination of detergent and acid washes and is then freeze dried. It is especially commercialized for reconstructive surgery, but clinical studies in wound care remain to be published.

3. GlyaDerm™ (Euro Skin Bank, Netherlands) is another acellular dermal collagen-elastin matrix, obtained by the treatment of glycerolized human donor skin with a low concentration of NaOH. The elastin matrix is not damaged by this manufacturing and preser vation method, which should lead to a more durable effect. [22,23] Additional advantages of glycerol preservation include inactivation of viruses and ease of storage and handling. GlyaDerm is provided by a non-governmental, non-profit organization, the Euro Skin Bank (the Netherlands) and is intended to be cost-effective, enabling widespread application.

4. SureDerm™ (Hans Biomed Corp. South Korea) is obtained by sequential treatments with dispase followed by Triton X-100. [24] The enzymatic treatment with dispase removes the epidermal layer. It is freeze-dried and stored at temperatures of 2°C to 8°C. SureDerm can be applied together with an one step split thickness skin graft, but there is a high risk of infection. Histologic examination showed that this product is completely absorbed within 4 months. [24]

5. CGDerm™ (Daewoong Bio Corp., Seoul Korea) is also an allograft derived from human skin. The epidermis and dermis are removed from the subcutaneous layer of the skin during the recovery procedure. The tissue is then processed using a sodium chloride solution and detergent to remove the epidermis and all viable dermal cells while maintaining the original dermal collagen matrix. The cells are removed to minimize inflammation or immunorejection at the surgical site. CGDerm™ is then treated in a disinfection solution that combines detergents with acidic and antiseptic reagents to further clean the tissue for sterility. Finally, it is freeze-dried, cut to size and packaged in a terminally sterilized double pouch and envelope. [25]

In a clinical report, an ADM with ultrathin autograft composite inhibited contraction and improved long-term cosmesis in patients with major burns. [26,27] A one-staged composite dermal and epidermal replacement was also reported with processed cadaver dermis and thin autograft for acute burn reconstructions. [28] Combined with AlloDerm® and a split-thickness skin graft, it can mimic a full-thickness skin graft providing a favorable long-term result. Thin autogenous skin graft or cultured keratocytes can be used over the ADM to provide permanent coverage. [27]

4. Clinical reports of ADM and split-thickness skin grafts

4.1. ADM and autograft for full thickness burn patients

The need to replace skin lost through injury is particularly crucial in extensively burned patients with limited donor site availability. Scar contracture with hypertrophy or joint contracture is common after 1:3~more meshed split thickness graftings. In full thickness burn patients, dermal component of ADM can prevent and reduce joint contracture and scar formation after skin graft surgery. Dermal component also reduce trans-epidermal water loss and erythema value than split thickness skin graft only group. [29] In the clinical report they used 1:3~6 meshed autograft as one-stage reconstruction method. [29] And in other reports comparing non-ADM graft only with 1:1.5 meshed skin graft and ADM graft with 1:1.5 mesh auto graft, skin elasticity was twice as high with ADM group in post operative day 60 and superior cosmesis without hypertrophic scarring in postoperative day 90. [5]

4.2. ADM and autograft for full-thickness scalp defects

In scalp wound patients which the calvaria is exposed, the use of flap is generally considered. However, in cases in which patients' general status is poor or vascular insufficiency is present, the use of flap becomes difficult. Treatment involved removal of the outer table of the skull and application of acellular human dermis (AlloDerm®). Then split-thickness skin graft was performed in a single phase split-thickness skin graft was performed in a single step. As compared with the flap,the use of AlloDerm® was technically simple and less time-consuming due to it being a single-step procedure. It is therefore effective in shortening the treatment period and securing excellent treatment outcomes. [30]

5. Problems using ADM and autograft

However, this process can be cumbersome when processed in single stage as a result of the need for serum imbibition and revascularization of separate layers of graft. So, a longer period of stabilization is required for revascularization to occur and to minimize the risk of graft failure. It is more true with unmeshed skin graft.

6. What is NPWT (Negative pressure wound therapy)?

Negative pressure wound therapy is a well-established form of treatment to enhance wound healing. It was first introduced by Argenta and Morykwas in 1997 and it has been used in a variety of conditions to reduce the size of wounds. [31,32] The mechanical force of negative pressure on wounds is known to augment local blood flow, reduce interstitial edema, reduce bacterial count, help retract the edges of the wound, and possibly affect the cellular activity and angiogenesis of the wound. [31-33,34] These factors together result in effective granulation and epithelization, successfully accelerating the healing of chronic wounds often seen in plastic and reconstructive, thoracic, orthopedic, and general surgical cases. [31,32,35-38]

6.1. NPWT for skin graft

The concept of using negative pressure wound therapy (NPWT) to secure a skin graft is not new. NPWT has been used instead of traditional dressing methods including bolster dressing or tie-over dressing. This technique provides near perfect contact between the graft and the recipient bed with a pressure equivalent to the negative pressure applied even on a complex curved anatomic areas. [39,40] NPWT minimizes shearing between the graft and wound bed and prevent formation of fluid and seroma also to promote proper contact between the graft and the recipient bed. Moreover, it may remove blood and exudates by negative pressure, minimizing the risk of hematoma as well as the risk of infection. [41] Improved microcirculation and increased tissue oxygen concentration also provide a desirable environment for graft survival. [42] NPWT also can be used to maximize graft take of full-thickness skin graft. [43] In treating the donor site of a radial forearm flap, Avery et al showed improved graft take without the need of splinting the arm, thereby reducing the morbidities and the length of hospital stay. [44]

Skin grafts typically fail because of shearing force over the graft skin or the development of a haematoma, seroma or infection underneath it. [45,46] The application of negative pressure contours the dressing materal so that it conforms to the wound surface. This stabilises the graft and helps prevent shearing and reduces the risk of haematoma and seroma formation, while helping to prevent contamination. Increased granulation facilitates revascularisation and attachment of the graft to the wound bed [35,36]. Numerous clinical studies have shown the successful use of NPWT in the management of skin and biomatrix grafts. [41,42,44,47,48]

A blinded, randomised controlled trial (RCT) investigated the effects of NPWT compared with standard bolster dressings over split-thickness skin grafts. Results showed that qualitative graft take was significantly better with NPWT as compared to standard bolster dressing ($P < 0\ 05$). NPWT over STSG improved the quality of the graft's appearance postoperatively, which may increase patient satisfaction. [49]

10-years retrospective review of 142 patients treated with an STSG in foot and ankle reconstructive surgeries also showed the effect of negative pressure wound therapy over skin graft. [48] Wound types included pressure, post-traumatic, and diabetic wounds, benign tumors, osteomyelitis, and other chronic ulcers. STSG patients received either NPWT (n = 87) or conventional therapy (n = 55) dressing. The results showed a significant difference in graft acceptance between the NPWT and conventional therapy groups. There were significantly fewer repeated graft and fewer complications, such as seroma, haematoma and infection, were observed

7. Negative pressure wound therapy for AlloDerm®–split-thickness skin graft

A retrospective study reports the use of negative pressure wound dressing with a simultaneous Acellular dermal matrix–split-thickness skin graft in resurfacing full-thickness defects and evaluates the efficacy over conventional tieover grafts. [50] A prospective study of 47 cases of skin defects treated by 1-stage allodermis and a split-thickness skin graft with NPWT showed that 97.8% graft take was noted at day 5 and the mean time until complete healing was 5.8 days. Statistically significant graft take (day 5) and time until complete healing was noted ($P < 0.05$). Good aesthetic and functional result mimicking a full-thickness skin graft was achieved. [50]

7.1. One-stage graft saves time and effort

Two-stage operation is common for wound coverage with ADM and autogenous skin graft. In most cases, use of acellular dermal matrix is followed by definitive coverage with skin graft at the second stage after the "take" of acellular dermal matix. [51] Negative pressure wound therapy make two-step procedure a single-stage operation. Negative pressure wound therapy over "composite of AMD and split-thickness skin" stabilizes the graft and remove hematoma or seroma under the skin and ADM. And it also facilitates revascularisation and attachment of the graft to the wound bed [35,36]. One-stage graft saves time and efforts of surgeon and patients by reducing operation time and dressing change.

8. Clinical applications

One-stage ADM and split-thickness skin graft can be applied to re-surface every types of wound with skin loss due to numerous etiologies including acute full thickness burns, acute trauma, chronic wounds, soft tissue defect with granulating bed and donor site of flap surgery which cannot be closed primarily.

8.1. Clinical cases

8.1.1. Case 1

A 71-year-old diabetic male was suffered from a diabetic foot. He had chronic renal failure on peritoneal dialysis. One month after percutaneous transluminal angioplasty of occlusions of superficial femoral artery, CGDerm™ and split thickness skin graft was done. After composite tissue graft, CuraVac® (400-600 μm pore size, Daewoong Pharm. CO. LTD., Seoul Korea) and portable suction device Curasys™ which provides cyclonic suction mode was applied for 10 days. Graft remain soft without any hypertrophic scar after 6 months. (Fig 1)

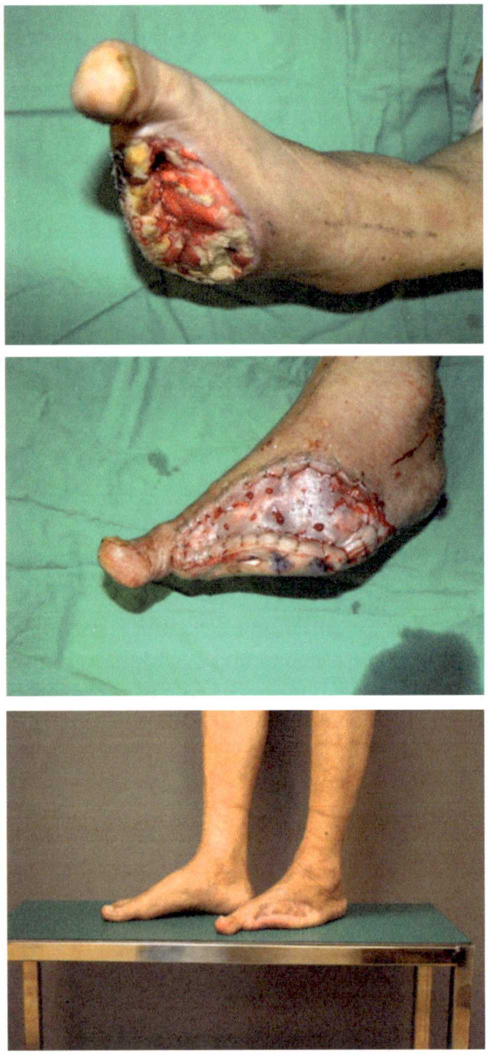

Figure 1. (Above) Before application of graft (Center) Just after grafting of CGDerm™ over granulating tissue (Below) 6 month following CGDerm™, split thickness skin graft and negative pressure wound therapy. After composite tissue graft, CuraVac® (400-600 μm pore size, Daewoong Pharm. CO. LTD., Seoul Korea) and portable suction device Curasys™ (Daewoong Pharm. CO. LTD., Seoul Korea) which provides cyclonic suction mode was applied for 10 days.

http://dx.doi.org/10.5772/53304

8.1.2. Case 2

A 74-year-old female was suffered from diabetic foot. After serial debridement, CGDerm™ and split thickness skin graft was done. After composite tissue graft, CuraVac® (400-600 μm pore size, Daewoong Pharm. CO. LTD., Seoul Korea) and portable suction device Curasys™ which provides cyclonic suction mode was applied for postoperative5 days. Graft maintained soft with minimal marginal hypertrophy. (Fig. 2)

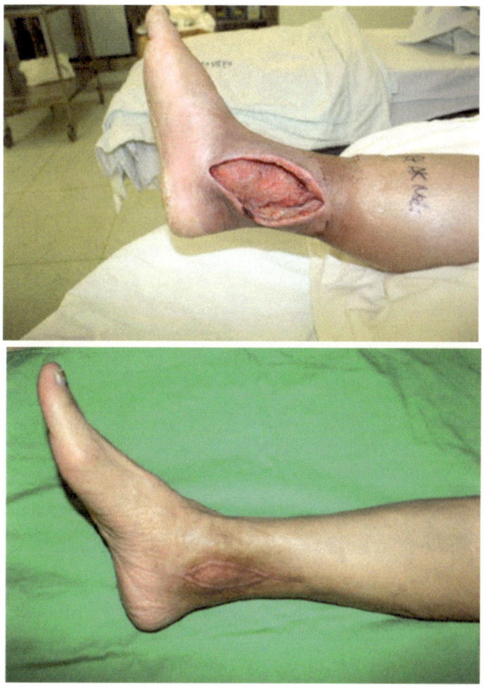

Figure 2. (Above) After debridement (Below) 2 months after CGDerm™, split thickness skin graft and negative pressure wound therapy. Wound remained soft without skin breakdown.

8.1.3. Case 3

A 60-year-old male had tonsil cancer. He underwent reconstruction with radial forearm free flap for oral cavity soft tissue defect. And donor site of radial forearm flap donor site was closed with CGDerm™, split thickness skin graft and negative pressure wound therapy. Graft remained soft without any ulceration. (Fig3)

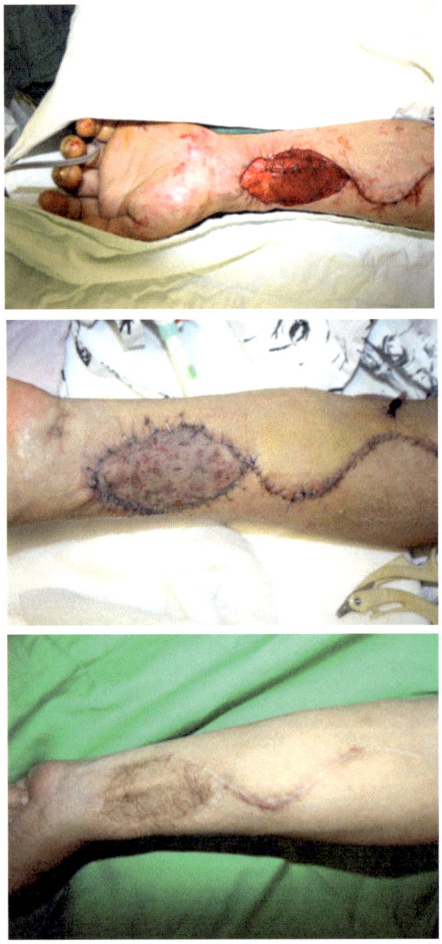

Figure 3. (Above) Before applying human acellular dermal matrix(ADM) (Center) 5 days after CGDerm™, split thickness skin graft and negative pressure wound therapy with CuraVac® and portable suction device Curasys™. Simple dressing was applied after removal of first negative pressure dressing. (Below) 2 years after skin graft

8.1.4. Case 4

A 57-year-old female underlying diabetes had necrotising fasciitis after consumption of seafood in overseas travel. She underwent serial debridement and CGDerm™, meshed split thickness skin graft and negative pressure wound therapy with CuraVac® was done. Wound remain soft without any hypertrophy after 8 months. (Fig 4.)

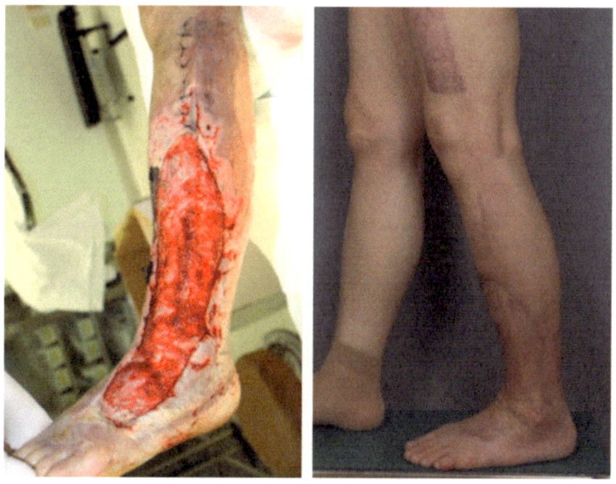

Figure 4. Left) After debridement and before skin grafting (Right) 8 month after AlloDerm® (Lifecell Corp., Branchburg, NJ) and thin split thickness skin graft. Wound remain soft without hypertrophy and ulceration.

9. Protocols

After adequate debridement of the wound bed, full range of the defect was covered with graftable ADM with 8~13/1000 inch thickness and fixed with minimal absorbable sutures after aseptical rehydrating of the implants with normal saline. Split-thickness skin graft was harvested from thigh or buttock region with a thickness of 8~12/1000 inches and a few slit incisions were made to promote removal of any fluid or blood. Skin was then sutured with non-absorbable suture or staplers to fix the graft to the bed and margin of the wound. Once the graft has been placed, a sterile open-cell, polyurethane ether foam containing PVC connection tubing is applied over the composite of AMD and split-thickness skin and sealed with occlusive dressing. A continuous or intermittent or cyclic negative pressure from 75mmHg to 125mmHg can be delivered by wall suction facilities or special suction device. Negative wound therapy was maintained for first 5 days and on the first opening of the wound, negative pressure dressing was stopped and minimal wound dressing was perform if needed. On day 5, you can confirm nearly complete take of composite tissue by checking adherence of graft and capillary refills. Additional dressing can be applied base on the needs.

10. Conclusion

Split-thickness skin added to acellular dermal matrix provides a sufficient amount of dermis to prevent contracture and promote better aesthetic outcome, and the negative pressure therapy ensured fast and complete take of the 2-layered composite graft. This option can be used to achieve healing mimicking a full-thickness skin graft without requiring large full-thickness donor sites.

11. Disclosure

The. senior author holds a co-patent for cyclic negative pressure wound therapy system and has given the rights to Daewoong Pharmaceutical Company.

Author details

Hyunsuk Suh and Joon Pio Hong

Department of Plastic Surgery, Seoul Asan Medical Center, University of Ulsan College of Medicine, Seoul, Korea

References

[1] JL. R. Greffes epidermiques. Bulletin de la Societe Imperiale de Chirurgie de Paris. 1869;10:51.

[2] Ragnell A. The secondary contracting tendency of free skin grafts; an experimental investigation on animals. Br J Plast Surg. 1952;5:6-24.

[3] Corps BV. The effect of graft thickness, donor site and graft bed on graft shrinkage in the hooded rat. Br J Plast Surg. 1969;22:125-133.

[4] Soejima K, Chen X, Nozaki M, Hori K, Sakurai H, Takeuchi M. Novel application method of artificial dermis: one-step grafting procedure of artificial dermis and skin, rat experimental study. Burns. 2006;32:312-318.

[5] Wainwright DJ. Use of an acellular allograft dermal matrix (AlloDerm) in the management of full-thickness burns. Burns. 1995;21:243-248.

[6] Costantino PD, Wolpoe ME, Govindaraj S, et al. Human dural replacement with acellular dermis: clinical results and a review of the literature. Head & neck. 2000;22:765-771.

[7] Kridel RW, Foda H, Lunde KC. Septal perforation repair with acellular human dermal allograft. Archives of otolaryngology--head & neck surgery. 1998;124:73-78.

[8] Bloemen MC, van Leeuwen MC, van Vucht NE, van Zuijlen PP, Middelkoop E. Dermal substitution in acute burns and reconstructive surgery: a 12-year follow-up. Plastic and reconstructive surgery. 2010;125:1450-1459.

[9] van Zuijlen PP, Vloemans JF, van Trier AJ, et al. Dermal substitution in acute burns and reconstructive surgery: a subjective and objective long-term follow-up. Plastic and reconstructive surgery. 2001;108:1938-1946.

[10] Oliver RF, Grant RA, Kent CM. The fate of cutaneously and subcutaneously implanted trypsin purified dermal collagen in the pig. British journal of experimental pathology. 1972;53:540-549.

[11] Fang CH, Robb EC, Yu GS, Alexander JW, Warden GD. Observations on stability and contraction of composite skin grafts: xenodermis or allodermis with an isograft overlay. The Journal of burn care & rehabilitation. 1990;11:538-542.

[12] Grillo HC, McKhann CF. The Acceptance and Evolution of Dermal Homografts Freed of Viable Cells. Transplantation. 1964;2:48-59.

[13] Oliver RF, Barker H, Cooke A, Stephen L. 3H-collagen turnover in non-cross-linked and aldehyde-cross-linked dermal collagen grafts. British journal of experimental pathology. 1982;63:13-17.

[14] Oliver RF, Barker H, Cooke A, Grant RA. Dermal collagen implants. Biomaterials. 1982;3:38-40.

[15] Walter RJ, Matsuda T, Reyes HM, Walter JM, Hanumadass M. Characterization of acellular dermal matrices (ADMs) prepared by two different methods. Burns. 1998;24:104-113.

[16] Jones I, Currie L, Martin R. A guide to biological skin substitutes. Br J Plast Surg. 2002;55:185-193.

[17] Kirsner RS, Falanga V, Eaglstein WH. The development of bioengineered skin. Trends in biotechnology. 1998;16:246-249.

[18] Livesey SA, Herndon DN, Hollyoak MA, Atkinson YH, Nag A. Transplanted acellular allograft dermal matrix. Potential as a template for the reconstruction of viable dermis. Transplantation. 1995;60:1-9.

[19] Rennekampff HO, Hansbrough JF, Woods V, Jr., Kiessig V. Integrin and matrix molecule expression in cultured skin replacements. The Journal of burn care & rehabilitation. 1996;17:213-221.

[20] Becker S, Saint-Cyr M, Wong C, et al. AlloDerm versus DermaMatrix in immediate expander-based breast reconstruction: a preliminary comparison of complication profiles and material compliance. Plastic and reconstructive surgery. 2009;123:1-6; discussion 107-108.

[21] Shores JT, Gabriel A, Gupta S. Skin substitutes and alternatives: a review. Advances in skin & wound care. 2007;20:493-508; quiz 509-410.

[22] Pirayesh A, Dur AH, Paauw NJ, et al. Evaluation of acellular dermis for closure of abdominal wall defects in a rat model. European surgical research. Europaische chirurgische Forschung. Recherches chirurgicales europeennes. 2008;41:346-352.

[23] Richters CD, Pirayesh A, Hoeksema H, et al. Development of a dermal matrix from glycerol preserved allogeneic skin. Cell and tissue banking. 2008;9:309-315.

[24] Takami Y, Matsuda T, Yoshitake M, Hanumadass M, Walter RJ. Dispase/detergent treated dermal matrix as a dermal substitute. Burns. 1996;22:182-190.

[25] Product information of CGDerm.

[26] Tsai CC, Lin SD, Lai CS, Lin TM. The use of composite acellular allodermis-ultrathin autograft on joint area in major burn patients--one year follow-up. Kaohsiung J Med Sci. 1999;15:651-658.

[27] Wainwright D, Madden M, Luterman A, et al. Clinical evaluation of an acellular allograft dermal matrix in full-thickness burns. The Journal of burn care & rehabilitation. 1996;17:124-136.

[28] Callcut RA, Schurr MJ, Sloan M, Faucher LD. Clinical experience with Alloderm: a one-staged composite dermal/epidermal replacement utilizing processed cadaver dermis and thin autografts. Burns. 2006;32:583-588.

[29] Yim H, Cho YS, Seo CH, et al. The use of AlloDerm on major burn patients: AlloDerm prevents post-burn joint contracture. Burns. 2010;36:322-328.

[30] Jung SN, Chung JW, Yim YM, Kwon H. One-stage skin grafting of the exposed skull with acellular human dermis (AlloDerm). The Journal of craniofacial surgery. 2008;19:1660-1662.

[31] Argenta LC, Morykwas MJ. Vacuum-assisted closure: a new method for wound control and treatment: clinical experience. Ann Plast Surg. 1997;38:563-576; discussion 577.

[32] Morykwas MJ, Argenta LC, Shelton-Brown EI, McGuirt W. Vacuum-assisted closure: a new method for wound control and treatment: animal studies and basic foundation. Ann Plast Surg. 1997;38:553-562.

[33] Jones SM, Banwell PE, Shakespeare PG. Advances in wound healing: topical negative pressure therapy. Postgraduate medical journal. 2005;81:353-357.

[34] Venturi ML, Attinger CE, Mesbahi AN, Hess CL, Graw KS. Mechanisms and clinical applications of the vacuum-assisted closure (VAC) Device: a review. American journal of clinical dermatology. 2005;6:185-194.

[35] Stone PA, Hass SM, Flaherty SK, DeLuca JA, Lucente FC, Kusminsky RE. Vacuum-assisted fascial closure for patients with abdominal trauma. The Journal of trauma. 2004;57:1082-1086.

[36] Tang AT, Okri SK, Haw MP. Vacuum-assisted closure to treat deep sternal wound infection following cardiac surgery. Journal of wound care. 2000;9:229-230.

[37] DeFranzo AJ, Marks MW, Argenta LC, Genecov DG. Vacuum-assisted closure for the treatment of degloving injuries. Plastic and reconstructive surgery. 1999;104:2145-2148.

[38] O'Connor J, Kells A, Henry S, Scalea T. Vacuum-assisted closure for the treatment of complex chest wounds. The Annals of thoracic surgery. 2005;79:1196-1200.

[39] Nakayama Y, Iino T, Soeda S. A new method for the dressing of free skin grafts. Plastic and reconstructive surgery. 1990;86:1216-1219.

[40] Stokes TH, Follmar KE, Silverstein AD, et al. Use of negative-pressure dressings and split-thickness skin grafts following penile shaft reduction and reduction scrotoplasty in the management of penoscrotal elephantiasis. Ann Plast Surg. 2006;56:649-653.

[41] Blackburn JH, 2nd, Boemi L, Hall WW, et al. Negative-pressure dressings as a bolster for skin grafts. Ann Plast Surg. 1998;40:453-457.

[42] Isago T, Nozaki M, Kikuchi Y, Honda T, Nakazawa H. Skin graft fixation with negative-pressure dressings. The Journal of dermatology. 2003;30:673-678.

[43] Landau AG, Hudson DA, Adams K, Geldenhuys S, Pienaar C. Full-thickness skin grafts: maximizing graft take using negative pressure dressings to prepare the graft bed. Ann Plast Surg. 2008;60:661-666.

[44] Avery C, Pereira J, Moody A, Gargiulo M, Whitworth I. Negative pressure wound dressing of the radial forearm donor site. International journal of oral and maxillofacial surgery. 2000;29:198-200.

[45] Hanasono MM, Skoracki RJ. Securing skin grafts to microvascular free flaps using the vacuum-assisted closure (VAC) device. Ann Plast Surg. 2007;58:573-576.

[46] Scherer LA, Shiver S, Chang M, Meredith JW, Owings JT. The vacuum assisted closure device: a method of securing skin grafts and improving graft survival. Arch Surg. 2002;137:930-933; discussion 933-934.

[47] Ward C, Ciraulo D, Coulter M, Desjardins S, Liaw L, Peterson S. Does treatment of split-thickness skin grafts with negative-pressure wound therapy improve tissue markers of wound healing in a porcine experimental model? The journal of trauma and acute care surgery. 2012;73:447-451.

[48] Blume PA, Key JJ, Thakor P, Thakor S, Sumpio B. Retrospective evaluation of clinical outcomes in subjects with split-thickness skin graft: comparing V.A.C.(R) therapy and conventional therapy in foot and ankle reconstructive surgeries. International wound journal. 2010;7:480-487.

[49] Moisidis E, Heath T, Boorer C, Ho K, Deva AK. A prospective, blinded, randomized, controlled clinical trial of topical negative pressure use in skin grafting. Plastic and reconstructive surgery. 2004;114:917-922.

[50] Kim EK, Hong JP. Efficacy of negative pressure therapy to enhance take of 1-stage allodermis and a split-thickness graft. Ann Plast Surg. 2007;58:536-540.

[51] Askari M, Cohen MJ, Grossman PH, Kulber DA. The use of acellular dermal matrix in release of burn contracture scars in the hand. Plastic and reconstructive surgery. 2011;127:1593-1599.

Chapter 5

Treatment of Leg Chronic Wounds with Dermal Substitutes and Thin Skin Grafts

Silvestro Canonico, Ferdinando Campitiello, Angela Della Corte, Vincenzo Padovano and Gianluca Pellino

Additional information is available at the end of the chapter

http://dx.doi.org/10.5772/51852

1. Introduction

Tissue repair is a natural process occurring any time the skin is injured. Repair is achieved through different successive phases: inflammation, formation of granulation tissue, formation of the extracellular matrix (ECM), and remodeling. ECM plays an important role in tissue regeneration representing the principal component of the dermal skin layer. The composition of ECM includes proteoglycans, hyaluronic acid, collagen, fibronectin and elastin. As well as providing a structural support for cells, some components of the ECM bind to growth factors, creating a reservoir of active molecules that can be rapidly mobilized following injury to stimulate cell proliferation and migration [1].

Acute wounds, such as traumatic or surgical wounds, generally require topical treatments leading to complete scar formation within 14 days. Treatment modalities, from topical treatments administered as a support for the physiological mechanisms of scarring to surgical repair with skin grafts, are usually chosen according to: dimension, location, and severity of the lesion; exposition of visceral or skeletal structures; age of the patient; risks related to other illnesses.

Some lesions, despite careful clinical examination, good physiopathologic classification, and adequate treatment (e.g. etiologic therapy, debridement and disinfection of the lesion, "humidification" of the surface) do not heal but achieve only temporary clinical improvement. Chronic wounds represent a state in which healing has stagnated.

Some studies showed that in chronic wounds the hyperproliferation of the edges inhibits the apoptosis of fibroblasts and keratinocytes [2]. Anomalies of the phenotype have also been associated with fibroblasts, such as altered morphology and a slower rate of proliferation [3,4]. Moreover, the fibroblasts obtained from chronic ulcers and cultivated in vitro have shown lesser response to exogenous application of growth factors such as platelet-derived growth factor [5,6]. This is because of fibroblasts being senescent and not truly responsive to stimuli, which would explain why the local application of growth factors to a chronic wound will not heal it [7,8]. In many chronic wounds, increased levels of inflammatory cells lead to elevated levels of proteases that seem to degrade the ECM components, growth factors, protein and receptors that are essential for healing [9].

Many surgical techniques and various types of advanced dressings are used for the treatment of these ulcers, assuming that the physiologic processes of tissue repair are competent and that the lesion can heal ''spontaneously''; this occurs quite frequently, but there are ulcers, usually defined as "complex", which do not heal within an acceptable timeframe, despite a correct diagnostic and therapeutic procedure, or relapse rapidly. This may be due to concomitant systemic pathologies (e.g. diabetes, immunodeficiency, cardiac failure) and/or to the presence of local factors (e.g. oedema, arterial or venous failure, infections) that inhibit the healing process. The lack of healing of the ulcer, even for years, affects the whole circumference of the leg, often involving deep structures such as aponeuroses and tendons. In such cases, a reconstructive surgical operation using skin grafts must always be considered, though it may also be difficult or likely to fail because of the position, width, and depth of the lesion(s).

When dealing with large full-thickness wounds of the lower limbs, the use of reconstructive operations with autologous skin grafting is widespread. Epidermis with a superficial part of the dermis is harvested with a dermatome from an undamaged skin donor site and applied to the full-thickness wound. Being applied to the wound, capillaries of the split skin graft (SSG) form anastomoses or "plug in" into the existing capillary network to provide nutrients for graft survival; this is referred to as graft "take". In the case of an extensive wound, donor sites are limited and in such cases, meshing techniques can be used meaning grafted skin is uniformly perforated and stretched to cover greater areas of the wound.

Nevertheless, full-thickness skin grafts require the taking of a sample, determining the creation of a wound that is itself deep and susceptible to complications such as infections and retractions of the scar, and precludes the use of the same site for the taking of further samples [10]. For this reason, one tends to prefer partial-thickness skin grafts, which in some cases may fail to attach and tend to retract, leading to unsatisfying results. That is for the most part due to the paucity or absence of derma in the partial-thickness skin grafts, as the dermal matrix plays a fundamental role in determining the success of a skin graft [11,12].

In these patients a new therapeutic perspective is "regenerative surgery" with the use of tissue-engineered products. In fact recognition of the importance of the ECM in wound healing has led to the development of wound products that aim to stimulate or replace the ECM. These tissue-engineered products comprise a reconstituted or natural collagen matrix that mimics the structural and functional characteristics of native ECM [13]. When placed into the wound bed, the three-dimensional matrix provides a temporary scaffold or support into

http://dx.doi.org/10.5772/51852

which cells can migrate and proliferate in an organized manner, leading to tissue regeneration and ultimately wound closure.

An ideal replacing skin product should principally contain these factors:

- the ECM;
- dermal fibroblasts;
- a semipermeable membrane between dermis and epidermis.

These components may act synergistically as part of a fully integrated tissue to protect the underlying tissues of a wound bed and to direct healing of the wound. Dermis containing fibroblasts could be necessary for the maintenance of the epidermal cell population.

All tissue-engineered skin substitute bioconstructs need to comply with three major requirements. They must be: safe for the patient, clinically effective, and convenient in handling and application. In general, such biomaterials must not be toxic, immunogenic or cause excessive inflammation, and should also have no or low level of transmissible disease risk. The biomaterial for skin reconstruction should be biodegradable, repairable and able to support the reconstruction of normal tissue, with physical and mechanical properties similar to those of the skin it replaces. It should provide pain relief, prevent fluid and heat loss from the wound surface and protect the wound from infection. It is also of great advantage if the skin substitute bioconstruct is cost-effective, readily available, user-friendly and with a long shelf life. No tissue-engineered skin replacement biomaterials currently available in commerce possess all the above-mentioned properties nor can any fully replace the functional and anatomical properties of the native skin. There are, however, a number of bioengineered skin-replacement products suitable for wound-healing purposes which are currently available to clinicians. In general, these tissue replacements only partially address skin functional requirements and surgeons tend to use different products to achieve specific purposes.

Tissue-engineered skin products may be either cellular, containing living cells (Table 1), or acellular, biologically inert (Table 2), and sourced from:

- Biological tissue: animal (e.g. equine/bovine/porcine); human (e.g. cadaveric skin); plant (e.g. containing oxidized regenerated cellulose/collagen)
- Synthetic materials
- Composite materials (containing two or more components, which may be biological or synthetic).

Different types of tissue-engineered products are available and confusion exists concerning the used terminology. Products may be classified as skin substitutes, xenografts, allografts or collagen dressings. "Skin substitutes" is an *umbrella term* for a group of products. Depending on individual characteristics, they may substitute or replace all or some components that compose normal skin (e.g. epidermis and/or dermis, cells and matrix). They can be bilayered, acellular or cellular, synthetic or biological and may consist of a synthetic epidermis and a collagen-based dermis to encourage formation of new tissue. In products with a synthetic epidermis, this may act as a temporary wound covering. Alternatively, these products may be described as *biological dressings* in that they serve as a protective wound cover. However, while most wound dressings need to be changed frequently, matrices provide a scaffold for tissue repair and therefore must remain in the wound for a sufficient length of time [23].

Product	Industry	Scaffold	Type	Cell Source	Indicated for Acute Wounds	Indicated for Chronic Wounds
Epicel®	Genzyme	Autologous keratinocytes, murine fibroblasts	Dermal +Epidermic	Autograft	+	+
Epidex®	Modex	Nitrocellulose	Epidermic	Autograft	+	+
MySkin	CellTRan Ltd.	Cultured Keratinocytes (subconfluent cell sheet)+silicon support layer with a specially formulated surface coating	Epidermic	Autograft	+	+
Cell Spray	Clinical Cell Culture	Non-/cultured Keratinocytes	Epidermic	Autograft	+	+
Bioseed-S	BioTissue Technologies	Cultured Keratinocytes (subconfluent cell sheet)+fibrin sealant	Epidermic	Autograft	+	+
Epibase	Laboratoires Genevirier	Cultured Keratinocytes (subconfluent cell sheet)	Epidermic	Autograft	+	+
Apligraf	Organogenesis Inc.	Cultured keratinocytes and fibroblast and bovine collagen	Dermal + Epidermic	Allograft	+	+
Orcel	Ortec International, Inc. NY	Cultured keratinocytes and fibroblast and bovine collagen sponge	Dermal + Epidermic	Allograft	+	+
PolyActive	HC Implants Bv, Leiden	Cultured keratinocytes and fibroblast in PEO/PBT	Dermal + Epidermic	Allograft	+	+

Product	Industry	Scaffold	Type	Cell Source	Indicated for Acute Wounds	Indicated for Chronic Wounds
Trancyte®	ATS	Silicon film, Nylon mesh, Porcine collagen+cultured neonatal fibroblast	Dermal	Allo- and synthetic graft	+	-
Dermagraft®	ATS	PLA/PGA+ ECM derived from fibroblast	Dermal	Allo - and synthetic graft	+	+
Graftskin	Organogenesis	Bovine collagen+ human keratinocytes and fibroblast	Dermal + Epidermic	Allograft	+	+
CSS®	Ortec International	Cross-linked bovine collagen and human cells	Dermal + Epidermic	Allograft	+	+
Keratinocytes crops	Lab. Ingegneria tessutale Università Milano	HYAFF®	Epidermic	Autograft	+	+
Laserskin®Autograft Hyalograft™ 3D	FAB	Cultured keratinocytes and fibroblast +HYAFF®	Dermal + Epidermic	Autograft	+	+

Table 1. Cellular-based tissue-engineered skin products currently in commerce

Engineered epidermal constructs with qualities similar to those of autologous skin have been used to facilitate repair of split-thickness wounds. Autologous cultured keratinocyte grafts have been used in humans since the 1980s. As a result there has been extensive experience with cultured epidermal grafts for the treatment of burns as well as other acute and chronic wounds [24]. Although they act as permanent wound coverage, since the host does not reject them, disadvantages include the two to three week time interval required before sufficient quantities of keratinocytes are available.

Cultured keratinocyte allografts were developed to overcome the need for biopsy and cultivation to produce autologous grafts and the long lag period between epidermal harvest and graft production. Cultured epidermal cells from both cadavers and adult donors have been used for the treatment of burns. Although a previous study showed that allografts made from neonatal foreskin keratinocytes were more metabolically active than those from cadaver, a recent study has shown that such allografts are immunogenic [16]. As an alternative, a chemically modified hyaluronic membrane acting as keratinocyte delivery system was developed. In this graft cells were delivered to the injury site via a biodegradable scaffold.

Product	Industry	Scaffold	Type	Cell Source	Indicated For Acute Wounds	Indicated For Chronic Wounds
Integra®	Integra Lifesciences-USA	Bovine type I collagen, chondrotin-6-sulfate, silicone	Dermal	Xeno - and synthetic graft	+	+
Matriderm®	Dr Suvelack Skin & Healthcare Ag-Germany	Bovine non-cross-linked lyofhilized collagen +elastinhydrolysate	Dermal	Xenograft	+	+
Unite Biomatrix®	TEVA-Pharmaceutical Industries LTD	Equin pericardium type I collagen	Dermal + Epidermic	Xenograft	+	+
Matristem™ Wound Care Matrix	ACELL Inc./Medline	Porcine urinary bladder matrix	Dermal	Xenograft	+	+
Ez-Derm™	AM Scientific / Brennen Medical	Porcine aldehyde cross-linked reconstituted dermal collagen	Dermal + Epidermic	Xenograft	+	+
Biodesign® (Surgisis®) Hernia Graft	Cook Medical	Porcine small intestine submucosa (SIS)	Dermal	Xenograft	+	-
Permacol	Covidien	Porcine acellular diisocyanite cross-linked dermis	Surgical biological implant for hernia & abdominal wall repair	Xenograft	+	-
CollaMend Implant	Davol Inc/Bard	Porcine Dermis	Surgical biological implantfor hernia & abdominal wall repair	Xenograft	+	-
XenMatrix Surgical Graft	Davol Inc/Bard	Porcine Dermis	Surgical biological implantfor hernia & abdominal wall repair	Xenograft	+	-
Puracol® Plus Microscaffold Collagen(Puracol Plus Ag)	Dr Suvelack Skin & Healthcare AG/ Medline	Bovine Collagen(plus antimicrobial Ag)	Surgical biological implantfor hernia & abdominal wall repair	Xenograft	+	-

Product	Industry	Scaffold	Type	Cell Source	Indicated For Acute Wounds	Indicated For Chronic Wounds
Biopad Collagen Wound Dressing	Euroresearch	Equine flexor tendon	Dermal	Xenograft	+	+
OASIS Wound Matrix	Healthpoint Ltd./ Cook Biotech, Inc	Porcine small intestine submucosa (SIS)	Dermal	Xenograft	+	+
Strattice™ Reconstructive Tissue Matrix	LifeCell	Porcine Dermis	Dermal	Xenograft	+	+
Endoform™ Dermal Template	Mesynthes	Propria submucosa layers of ovine forestomach	Dermal	Xenograft	+	-
Veritas Collagen Matrix	Synovis Orthopedic and Woundcare	Bovine pericardium	Surgical biological implant for abdominal wall repair& breast reconstruction	Xenograft	+	-
Primatrix™ Dermal Repair Scaffold	TEI Biosciences	Fetal bovine dermis	Dermal	Xenograft	+	-
SurgiMend®/ SurgiMend®Hernia Repair Matrix	TEI Biosciences	Fetal bovine dermis	Surgical biological implantfor hernia & abdominal wall repair	Xenograft	+	-
Alloderm®	KCL/ LifeSciences	Human skin tissue	Dermal	Allograft	+	-
Hyalomatrix PA®	FAB	Membrane HYAFF® layered on silicon	Dermal	Allo - and synthetic graft	+	-
Biobrane®	Smith&Nephew	Silicon film, nylon fabric, porcine collagen	Dermal + Epidermic	Xeno - and synthetic graft	+	+
Suprathel®	Healtcare	Polylattic acid	Epidermic	Xenograft	+	+
Jaloskin®	FAB	HYAFF11	Epidermic	Xenograft	+	-
Graftygen Epidermis®	TEVA	Mycrolose	Epidermic	Xenograft	+	+
Graftygen Derma®	TEVA	Collagen (3D)	Dermal	Allograft	+	+

Product	Industry	Scaffold	Type	Cell Source	Indicated For Acute Wounds	Indicated For Chronic Wounds
Neoform™	Mentor	Human dermis	Dermal	Allograft	+	+
Pelnac Standard/ Pelnac Fortified	Gunze Limited, Medical Material Center	Silicone/silicone fortified with silicone gauze TRX,Porcine tendon –derived atenocollagen	Dermal	Xeno - and synthetic graft	+	-
SureDerm Acellular	Hans Biomed Corporation	Human acellular lyofilized dermis	Dermal	Allograft	+	+
GraftJacket	Wright Medical Technology, Inc.	Human acellular pre-meshed dermis	Dermal	Allograft	+	-
Karoderm	Karocell Tissue Engineering AB	Human acellular dermis	Dermal	Allograft	+	+
AllomaxSurgical Graft	Davol Inc/Bard	Human acellular dermis	Surgical biological implant for hernia & abdominal wall	Allograft	+	-
Dermamatrix Acellular Dermis	MusculoskeletalTran splant Foundation/ Synthes CMF	Human acellular dermis	Surgical biological implant for hernia & abdominal wall	Allograft	+	-
FlexHD Acellular Hydrated Dermis	MusculoskeletalTran splant Foundation/ Ethicon	Human acellular dermis	Dermal	Allograft	+	-
Terudermis	Olympus Terumo Biomaterial	Silicone, bovine lyophilized cross-linked collagen sponge made of heat-denatured collagen	Dermal	Xeno - and synthetic graft	+	-

Table 2. Acellular tissue-engineered skin products in commerce.

Keeping in mind that good skin regeneration requires an appropriate dermal layer, allografts (containing dermis) from other sources have been used for many years, although they provide only temporary coverage due to their tendency to induce acute inflammation. However, this skin can be chemically treated to remove the antigenic epidermal cellular elements and has been used alone or in combination with cultured autologous keratinocytes for closure of various chronic wounds and burns. In spite of these modifications, allogeneic grafts, when compared with autologous grafts, have been shown to promote lower percentages of re-epithelization and excessive wound contraction [17].

Acellular matrices may be either animal- or human-derived, with all cells removed during manufacture, or they may be either synthetic or composite, if cells are naturally not present from the outset. These matrices or tissue scaffolds provide a collagen structure for tissue remodeling, while the removal of viable cells aims to minimize or prevent an inflammatory or immunogenic response [18]. A matrix may be described as a tissue scaffold in that it provides a supporting structure into which cells can migrate. However, it should be noted that a scaffold does not have to be a matrix (e.g. it does not interact with cells to the same degree as a matrix). For example, fibronectin may act as a matrix, but it is not necessarily a scaffold; similarly, polyglactin may act as a scaffold, but it is not a matrix [14].

Given current knowledge, the ideal acellular matrix is one that most closely approximates the structure and function of the native ECM it is replacing.

An acellular composite skin graft containing bovine collagen and chondroitin-6-sulfate with an outer silicone covering was developed in the 1980s. After placement on the wound, the acellular dermal component recruits the host dermal fibroblasts while undergoing simultaneous degradation. About two or three weeks later, the silicone sheet is removed and covered with an autograft. This composite graft has been used successfully to treat burns [19]. However, these constructs cannot be used in patients who are allergic to bovine products.

Another type of dermal substitute consists of an inner nylon mesh in which human fibroblasts are embedded, together with an outer silicone layer. After an appropriate time, fibroblasts are laid in the final product by freeze-thawing. Prior to that time, fibroblasts produce autologous collagen, matrix proteins and cytokines, all of which promote wound healing by the host. This product has been used successfully as temporary wound coverage after excision of burn wounds, until the appearance of the modified product on the market. The new graft contains a biodegradable polyglactin mesh, in which fibroblasts retain viability, instead of the nylon mesh. The use of this dermal substitute has had limited success in the treatment of diabetic foot ulcers, owing largely to its inability to form stable adhesions with the final epidermal graft [20].

Full-thickness wounds involve the loss of both the epidermal and dermal layers of the skin. To treat such extensive wounds, a two-layer skin composite was developed consisting of a collagen sponge containing dermal fibroblasts covered with epidermal cells. A subsequent amendment containing type I bovine collagen and live allogeneic human skin fibroblasts and keratinocytes has been developed. It has been used successfully in surgical wounds and venous ulcers [21]. In a multicenter trial, this product produced accelerated healing of chronic non-healing venous stasis ulcers when compared to standard compressive therapy [22].

Several other composite skin substitutes combining dermal and epidermal elements have been developed. Composite cultured skin composed of an overlay of stratified neonatal keratinocytes on fibroblasts embedded in distinct layers of bovine type I collagen is currently being evaluated in clinical trials for the treatment of burns.

Currently the acellular matrix products differ mainly in the source of cells and tissue materials and methods used during manufacture. A variety of animal- and human-derived products are available (Table 2), as in the reference [14].

Products derived from animal sources (xenografts) are developed by harvesting living tissue (e.g. dermis, small intestine submucosa, pericardium, etc) from various donor animals (e.g. porcine, equine or bovine) at different stages of development. The tissue materials are subsequently processed to remove the cells (decellularization), leaving the collagen matrix. Products derived from animal sources may either consist of the tissue scaffold only (e.g. Unite® BioMatrix Collagen Wound Dressing, Synovis) or may be combined with synthetic materials to create a composite product (e.g. INTEGRA® Bilayer Matrix Wound Dressing, Integra LifeSciences).

Products derived from human sources, i.e. donated human cadaver skin allografts, undergo various processes to remove the cells and deactivate or destroy pathogens (e.g. AlloDerm®, Lifecell; GraftJacket®, Wright Medical).

The mechanisms by which acellular matrices promote wound healing remain to be elucidated and there is ample scope for further research. It is known from the literature that chronic or hard-to-heal wounds are characterized by a disrupted or damaged ECM that cannot support wound healing. Treatment strategies that are designed to replace the absent or dysfunctional ECM may be beneficial [9]. As a result, there is renewed interest in collagen-based advanced wound care products.

In chronic wounds, there is an excess of MMPs and reduced growth factor activity. Together these result in the degradation of the ECM. For wound healing to occur the balance between protease and growth factor activity needs to be adjusted [9]. Research has demonstrated that topically applied collagen-based products can initiate wound healing by binding to and inactivating harmful proteases, while encouraging angiogenesis and formation of granulation tissue [23].

Current information about the mode of action of acellular matrices is largely based on preclinical data, mainly from research focusing on a porcine-derived small intestinal submucosa (SIS) wound matrix. These data show that matrices may:

- Act as a scaffold to support cell ingrowth and granulation tissue formation [24]
- Have receptors that permit fibroblasts to attach to the scaffold [25]
- Stimulate angiogenesis [26]
- Act as a chemoattractant for endothelial cells1 [27]
- Contain/protect growth factors1 [28].

When used as an implant, the acellular matrix appears to be fully incorporated into the wound. However, when used in a chronic wound, the matrix is eventually displaced and is not fully incorporated. As such, the role of acellular matrices in chronic wounds is not fully understood. It has been suggested that they act as a biological cover that modulates the wound environment to promote normal wound healing.

In the references [29,30] the Authors suggested the mode of action of collagen-based acellular matrix products:

- Chronic wounds contain high levels of MMPs which can:
- Degrade the ECM and growth factors
- Increase inflammatory response
- Reduce cell responsiveness in the wound
- Delay wound healing
- An acellular matrix that closely resembles native ECM may act as a scaffold for:
- MMPs to bind to and break down collagen in the product
- Epithelial cells, fibroblasts and vascular endothelial cells to migrate into and proliferate
- Reduced levels of MMPs to be released back into wound as collagen matrix breaks down, rebalancing protease and growth factor levels in the wound
- Enhanced wound healing environment, where matrix has been replaced by new collagen with remodeling of ECM.

Acellular matrices should be considered in wounds that are unresponsive to traditional wound management modalities or present as a complex surgical wound. Factors to consider will be dependent on the wound type, underlying etiology, patient suitability and treatment goal. In a non-healing chronic wound (e.g. diabetic foot ulcer), for example, an acellular matrix may be selected to replace the damaged ECM, fill the defect and optimize the wound environment for healing.

In the reference [14] the Authors have proposed an algorithm for application of acellular matrices in a chronic wound, as reported in Table 3. Previous studies have shown that reduction in the area of the chronic wound during the first four weeks of treatment is a predictor of complete healing at 12 weeks [31]. If no improvement is seen at this time, there should be further evaluation of the patient and current treatment strategy.

Our own experience in the treatment of complex leg ulcers is prevalently related to the use of a dermal matrix that stimulates the production of endogenous collagen, determining the constitution of a functional dermis (Integra Dermal Regeneration Template). It is a "semibiological implant" consisting of a two-layered membrane. The thin external pellicle, in silicone, allows for the immediate closure of the wound, controlling the loss of fluids and proteins, providing it with mechanical and antibacterial protection [32]. The internal layer consists of a porous matrix composed of type 1 collagen from bovine tendons and from glycosaminoglycan (chondroitin-6-sulfate) that produces a histoinductive and histoconductive action on the mesenchyme, leading to the formation of normal derma. The collagen represents only its structural base, whereas the chondroitin (8% of its weight) confers its principal properties on the matrix. The glycosaminoglycans, such as hyaluronan, dermatan, and keratan, are important in the constitution of the ECM and in the regulation of the cellular development and differentiation. They are predominant in the embryonic tissue and accumulate in fetal wounds, which repair through regeneration without inflammation or scarring in fibrosis [33,34]. The chondroitin, moreover, masks the sites of binding on the collagen, preempting platelet adhesion and the consequent inflammation [35].

Assessment of patient and wound to establish diagnosis and suitability	
Meets criteria (e.g. diabetic, venous, vasculitic, trauma wound	Does not meet criteria (e.g. severe arterial disease). Do not apply matrix
Address intrinsic problems and control infection	Unable to control infection. Do not apply matrix
Ensure appropriate wound bed preparation to maximize healing potential	Wound bed is not viable. Do not apply matrix
Consider options for treatment (including acellular/cellular matrix, growth factors, etc)	
Wound bed is viable and infection controlled Apply acellular matrix Consider adjunctive therapies, for example: NPWT to control exudates, topical antimicrobial to control infection, compression to control oedema	
Review at 7 days Address any complications, e.g. apply new matrix if product is displaced Continue to address intrinsic problems and control infection Change secondary dressing	
Continue to observe	
Re-epithelization and wound healing	

Table 3. Algorithm for application of acellular matrices in a chronic wound [14]

When the Integra is applied to a lesion, the inflammation stops because the matrix not only seems to be invisible to the platelets and inflammatory leucocytes, but also seems to be rec-

http://dx.doi.org/10.5772/51852

ognized as self. One does not find microscopic inflammatory infiltrates or clinical signs of inflammation. Pain is often absent after the application of Integra, and perilesional erythema and oedema disappear quickly. The hypotheses that explain the phenomenon can be summarized as follows. The lack of adhesion of the platelet anticipates the acute inflammation, and the artificial dermis confines the lesion, eliminating local exposition, desiccation, bioburden, and similar secondary damage. The chondroitin matrix is sufficiently similar to normal tissue such that the leukocytes and lymphocytes cross the matrix without recognizing any abnormality and without thus producing any defensive reaction [36]. In summary, when the dermal matrix is imposed on a skin lesion, all of the factors that cause damage are stopped, and from a functional perspective, regeneration is the only available response.

Four distinct phases of regeneration of the dermis were recognized in the period of attachment of the dermal matrix (imbibition, migration of the fibroblasts, new vascularization, and maturation with remodeling) without the presence of nerve endings or elastic fibers. The new collagen is therefore indistinguishable from the normal collagen of the dermis [37].

Compared with the healing obtained with autotransplantation of skin, that achieved using grafting with Integra are also found to be clinically better and comparable with normal skin [38].

Brought into clinical use in 1981, Integra was first used for the treatment of burns, predominantly those that were deep and covering a large area [39-41]. Subsequently, its use was extended to reconstructive surgery on strongly retracted scars [42]. It was found to be particularly useful in covering deep structures such as periosteum and tendons.

Before the application of Integra, the wounds are to be cleaned and disinfected with antibiotic drugs and advanced dressings during periodic close examinations. Once surgery is planned, the choice of local or epidural anesthesia is based on the number and dimensions of the ulcers treated. First, surgical debridement of the lesion(s) is performed aiming to reduce the bacterial ratio, level the deep surface of the ulcer, and regulate its edges: we perform surgical cleansing and the preparation of the margins of the ulcers with a hydrosurgery system. To facilitate and improve modeling and attachment of the dermal matrix, its margins are modeled with scissors to fit perfectly and fixed to the skin with metal clips or topical skin adhesive. Petroleum jelly dressing and compressed multilayer bandages are applied on the wound. Postoperative treatment consists of antibiotic and analgesic drugs; analgesic therapy is provided according to the level of patient pain.

The first postoperative medication is administered after 8 days, the metallic clips (if present) are removed, and the antibiotic therapy suspended. Usually at the first follow-up a notable reduction of moisture and surrounding oedema is ascertained. The patients are then treated in the outpatient clinic with silver dressings every 5 to 7 days, based on the degree of moisture.

After 21 days, the attachment of the artificial dermis is tested. Usually the dermal matrix is completely integrated with the guest tissue, having formed a new homogeneous and living derma. The next skin-graft operation is planned and the patient is readmitted for surgery. The epidermis (0.15–0.25 mm thick) is extracted with dermatome from the front part of the thigh, treated with mesh graft, and fixed on the lesion with metal clips. The wounds are covered again with petroleum jelly gauze and compressive bandages, and the previous antibiotic therapy is recommenced. After 8 days, the first follow-up is planned for the removal of the clips and the first test of the attachment of the graft. This is covered again with silver medications, and antibiotics are stopped. Further checks are planned weekly until the ulcer is completely healed. After that, a monthly follow-up is planned.

We performed a prospective observational study from April 2005 to June 2011 enrolling patients with leg ulcers that were not healing for at least 1 year. The ulcers were at least 100 cm^2 in area (in the case of multiple ulcers of the same limb, the overall surface area was taken into account) and at least 3 mm deep over at least 50% of the surface area. Patients who had an obstructive arterial disease were excluded from the study. The dimensions and depth of the ulcers were measured using the Visitrak digital apparatus (Smith & Nephew Medical Limited, Hull, UK). For all patients, there was a preliminary culture on the biopsy of the lesion. All patients' wounds were cleaned and disinfected with antibiotic drugs and advanced dressings during periodic close examinations at the outpatient clinic of the operating Unit.

Once surgery was planned, the patients were informed about the procedure and gave their written consent. The choice of anaesthetic (local or epidural) was based on the number and dimensions of the ulcers to be treated. First, surgical debridement of the lesion(s) was performed aiming to reduce the level of bacteria, level the deep surface of the ulcer, and establish the periphery of the dermal matrix to facilitate and improve its modeling and attachment. The matrix was modeled with scissors to fit perfectly and was applied by fixing the edges of the matrix to the skin with metal clips or topical skin adhesive (2-octil-cyanoacrylate, Dermabond, Ethicon Inc., Somerville, NJ). The medication was applied with petroleum jelly gauze and compressed multilayer bandage. Postoperative treatment consisted of antibiotic and analgesic drugs. Analgesic therapy was provided according to the level of pain that the patient reported. The same nurse evaluated pain using a 10 cm visual analogical scale (VAS) from 0 (no pain) to 10 (maximum pain) before the operation and on postoperative day third, eighth, and fifteenth. The first postoperative medication was administered after 8 days, the metallic clips (if present) were removed and the antibiotic therapy suspended. The patients were then treated in the outpatient clinic with silver dressings every 5 to 7 days, based on the degree of the exudates. After 21 days, the attachment of the artificial dermis was tested, and in positive cases, the patient was readmitted for the surgical application of a "thin" skin graft. The epidermis (0.15-0.25 mm thick) was extracted with dermatome from the front part of the thigh, treated with mesh graft, and fixed on the lesion with metal clips. The lesions were covered again with petroleum jelly gauze and compressive bandages, and the previous antibiotic therapy was recommenced. After 8 days, the first follow-up was planned for the removal of the clips and the first test of the attachment of the graft. This was covered again with the silver medication, and antibiotic therapy was stopped. Further checks were planned weekly until the ulcer was completely healed. After that, a monthly follow-up was planned. Independent experts photographically documented all of the treatment phases in all cases.

Three-hundred eighty-three consecutive patients were admitted to the study: 109 were male (28.45%) and 274 were female (71.54%). The median age was 64 (range 37–90) years. The ulcers were classified according to their etiology: 135 were lymphovenous (35.24%) (Figures 1-6), 87 venous (22.71%), 69 due to vasculitis (18.01%), 38 cancerous (9.92%), 29 posttraumatic (7.57%), 18 neuropathic (4.69%) (Figures 7-11), three were due to chemotherapy (0.78%) one was the consequence of laser therapy (0.26%), and one was the consequence of surgery (0.26%). In 117 patients (30.05%), the ulcers were located on both legs and were treated contemporaneously with an identical technique, for a total of 646 limbs treated. All of the ulcers were infected and required targeted antibiotic therapy. The germs identified were Staphylococcus aureus (50.0%), Pseudomonas aeruginosa (50.0%) Enterobacter cloacae (15.4%), S. epidermis (15.4%), Proteus mirabilis (7.6%), and Streptococcus Beta-Haemoliticus (7.6%). Sometimes more than one type of germ was found in the same patient. At the preoperative evaluation, all of the patients complained of continuous and intense pain, ranging from a minimum of 6 to a maximum of 10 (average 7.8) on the VAS scale. In 169 patients (44.1%) who had good cleansing of the ulcer, the Integra was applied using a local anaesthetic, fixing it to the skin with the Dermabond after debridement of brushing and washing with a physiological solution. For the other 214 patients (55.8%), 133 (58.8%) of whom had bilateral lesions and 71 (41.2%) exposed aponeuroses or tendons, the operation was performed using an epidural anaesthetic. In all of these cases, the surgical cleansing and the preparation of the margins of the ulcers were performed using a hydro-surgery system, and the Integra was attached with metal clips.

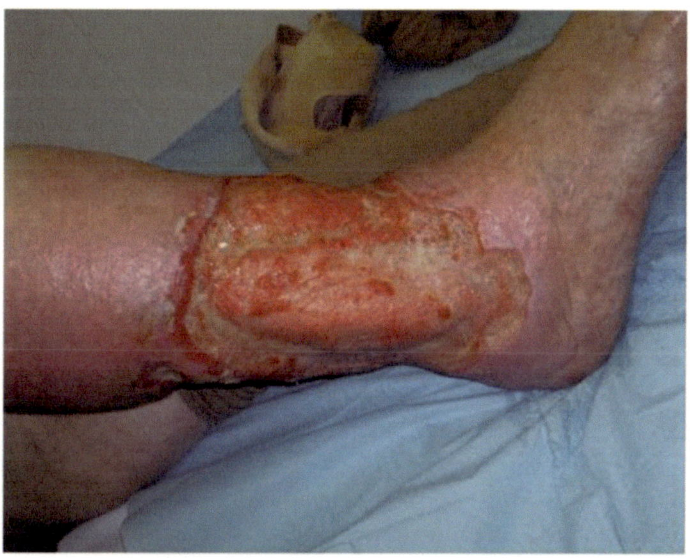

Figure 1. Lympho-venous ulcer of the right leg lasting for more than 12 months.

At the follow-up on the third day after surgery, all patients reported a substantial reduction in local pain (median VAS 3.8, range 1–6) which allowed 88 (23.1%) patients to suspend the analgesic therapy. At the follow-up on the eighth day, there was a further reduction in the level of pain (median VAS 2.8, range 1–4). By the third check on the 15th day, the pain reported had reduced further (median VAS 1.7, range 0–3) and all of the patients were able to stop the analgesic therapy.

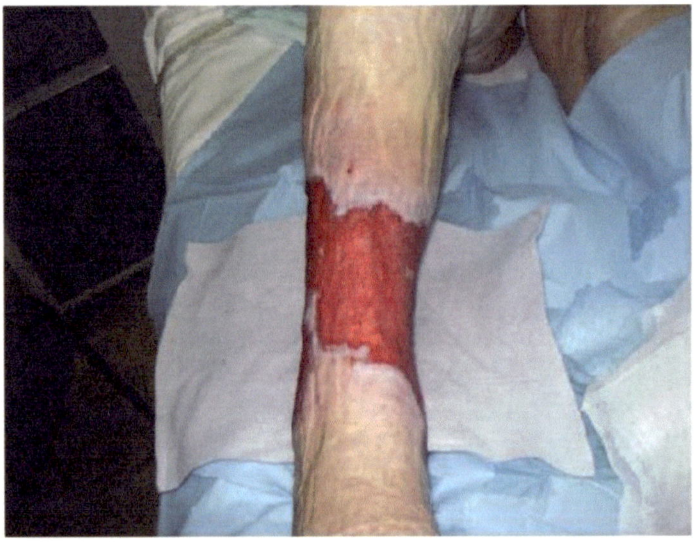

(a)

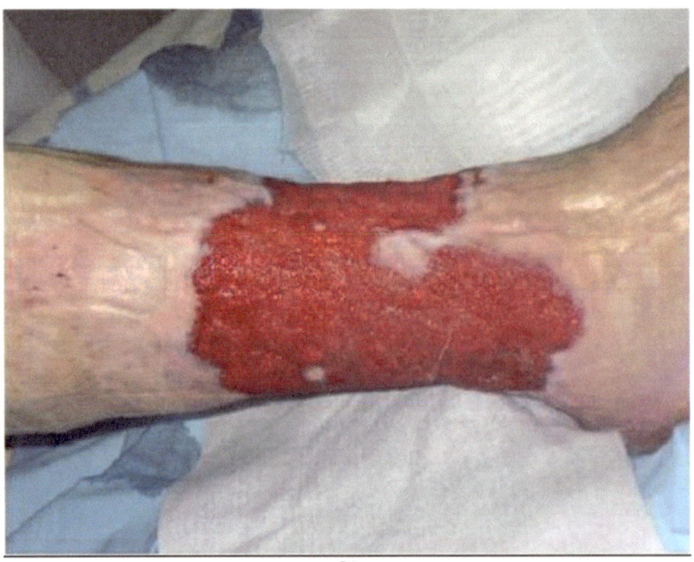

(b)

Figure 2. a,b) The same case as figure 1. View after outpatient treatment of the wound and its debridement with Versajet hydrosurgery.

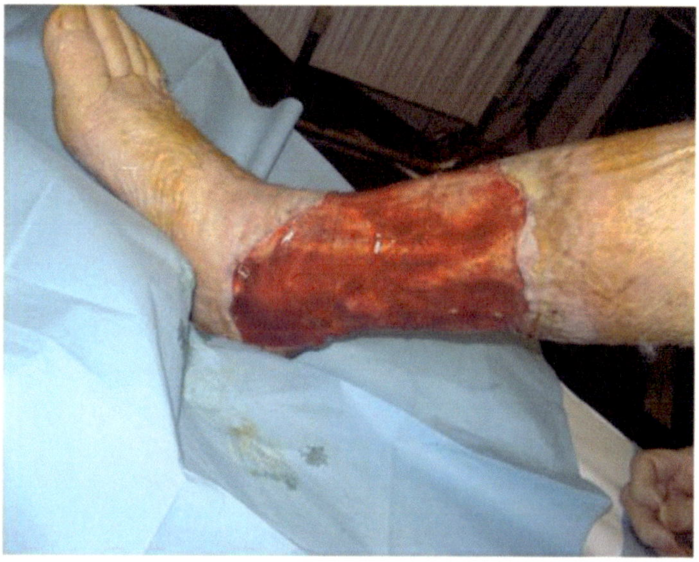

Figure 3. The same case as figure 1. View of the ulcer 1 week after the application of the Integra dermal substitute. The brightness of the silicone layer is evident.

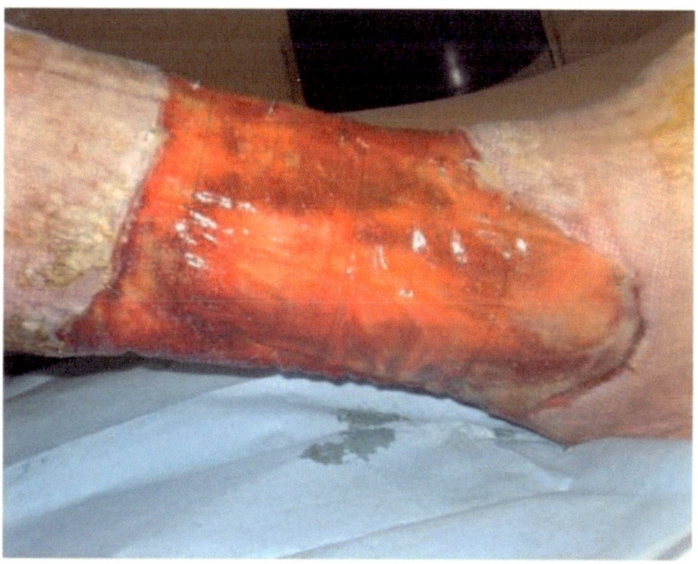

Figure 4. The same case as figure 1. View of the ulcer 3 weeks after the application of the Integra dermal substitute. The new dermis is completely reconstructed, and the wound is ready for the epidermis skin graft.

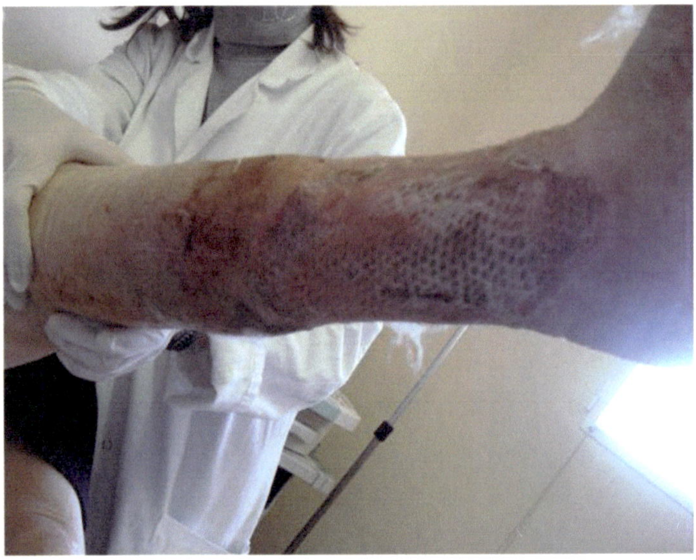

Figure 5. The same case as figure 1. View of the wound at the end of thin skin graft

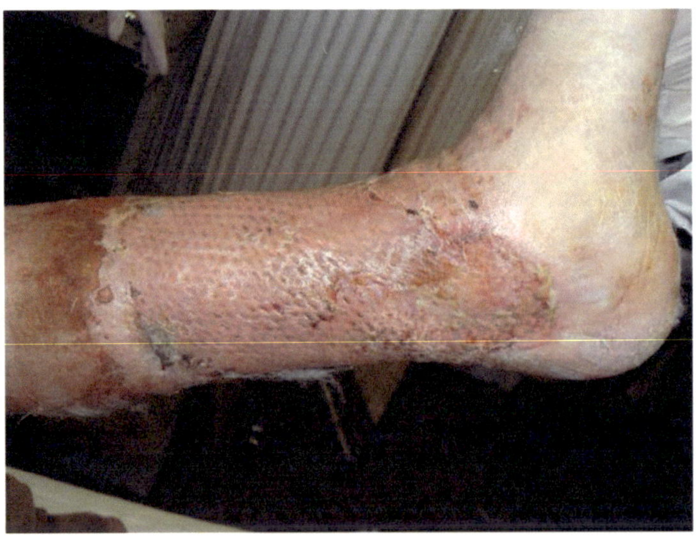

Figure 6. The same case as figure 1. View of the wound 2 weeks after thin skin graft, which is completely attached.

http://dx.doi.org/10.5772/51852

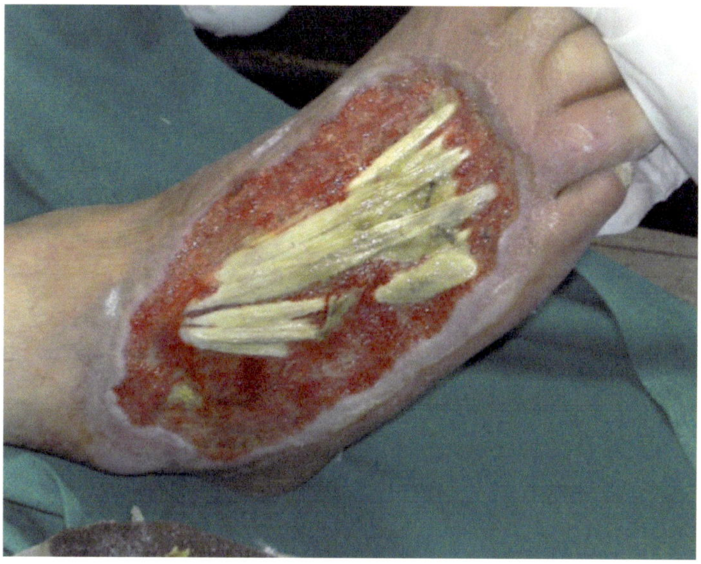

Figure 7. Neuropathic ulcer of the right leg.

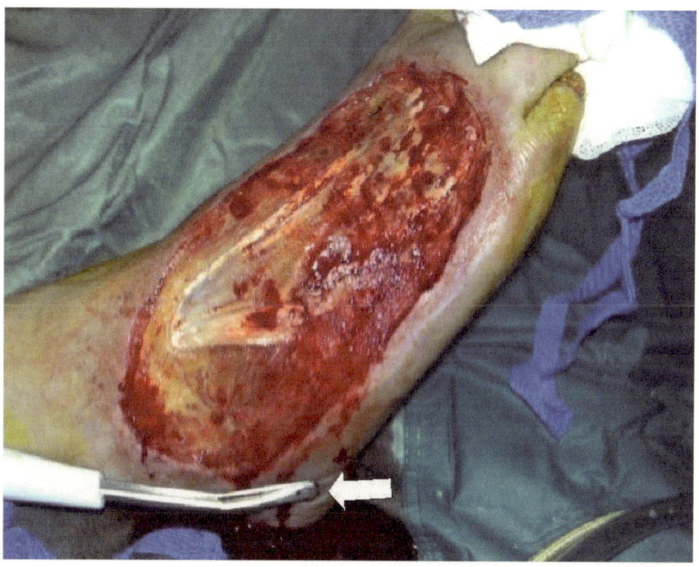

Figure 8. The same case as figure 7. Intraoperatory view during wound debridement with Versajet hydrosurgery (arrow).

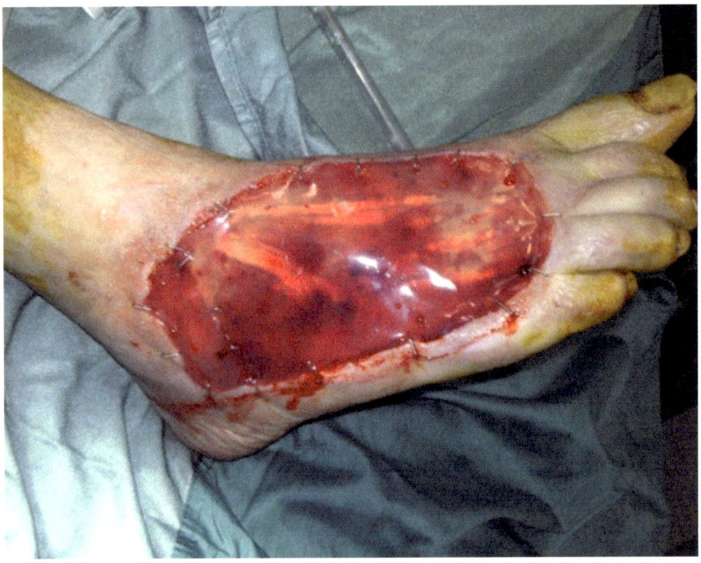

Figure 9. The same case as figure 7. View of the ulcer 1 week after the application of the Integra dermal substitute.

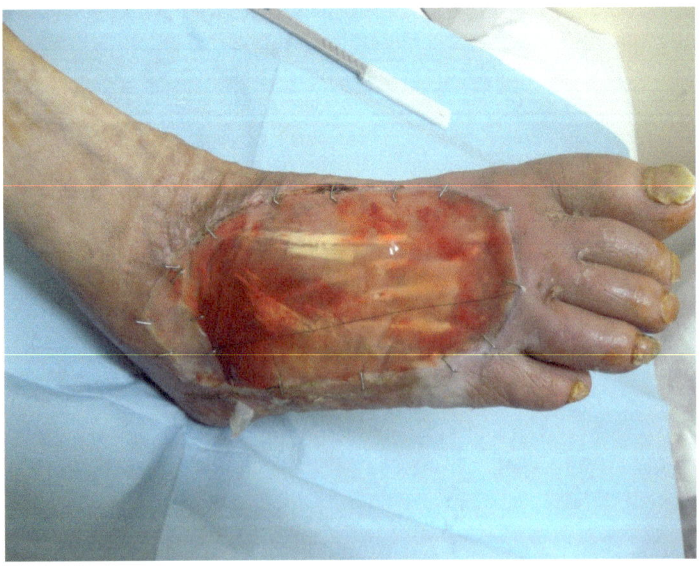

Figure 10. The same case as figure 7. View of the ulcer 3 weeks after the application of the Integra dermal substitute.

http://dx.doi.org/10.5772/51852

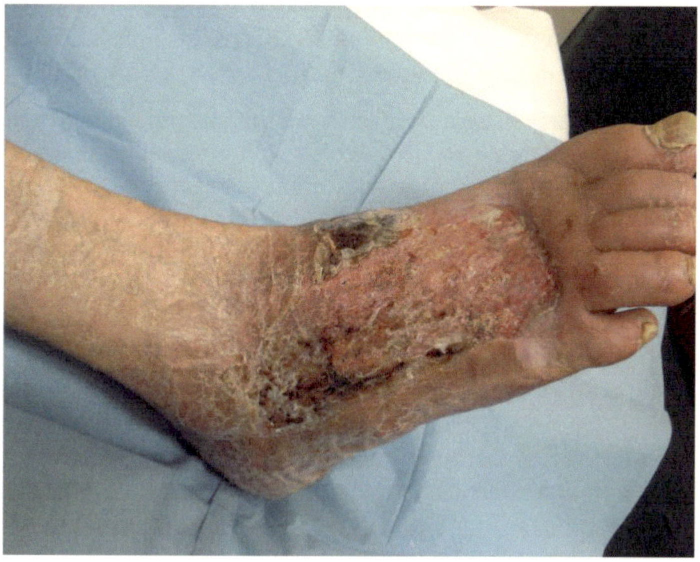

Figure 11. The same case as figure 7. View of the wound 2 weeks after thin skin graft..

In all patients, at the first follow-up, a notable reduction in the exudate and the perilesional oedema was ascertained. After 2 weeks the progressive substitution of granulation tissue with new yellow or gold derma became evident through the layer of silicone. Only in 50 cases (7.7%) was it necessary to partially remove the layer of silicone because some areas showed abundant yellowish exudates under the lamina. The neodermis, remaining thus uncovered and without protection, was covered with hydrofibrous and silver dressings, although that did not prevent, even in these patients, the complete formation of the neodermis.

At the check on the 21st day, in all cases, the dermal matrix was completely integrated with the guest tissue, having formed a new homogeneous and living derma, and the next skin-graft operation was planned.

In 339 patients (88.5%) the attachment of the skin graft was complete, whereas in 44 patients (11.5%) it was partial but nevertheless larger than 70% of the surface, but, even in these cases, complete healing of the lesion was achieved within 4 weeks at the most. The definitive result was therefore the complete healing of all of the lesions. All of the patients were examined in follow-up visits for a minimum of 3 months; none suffered from an ulcerous recurrence.

According to our experience, in all of the patients suffering from deep and wide leg ulcers, the use of Integra dermal matrix allowed for the complete refilling of the loss of tissue, with covering of the uncovered anatomical structures such as tendons and aponeuroses, fast and occasionally immediate disappearance of pain in almost all cases, and rapid regeneration of a permanent dermis. The quality, flexibility, and elasticity of the neodermis confirmed the difference from the scar tissue and its similarity to the normal dermis, resulting in better mechanical resistance of the neodermis and fewer tendencies toward hypertrophy of the scar.

This therefore allows the application of a thin epidermal skin graft that requires a secure and faster attachment than a total- or partial-thickness skin graft but also consistent improvement in terms of functional and aesthetic results.

Future directions and research lines in chronic wounds treatment will have to deal with several issues. Concerning tissue-engineered products for skin substitution, these have been associated with improved survival rate and quality of life in patients with extensive burns [43]. However, despite promising results have been reported in clinical trial with products based on autologous cultured keratinocytes and fibroblasts [44], actually these can only serve as a bridge to autografting rather than being suitable for fully replace damaged skin [43,45].

Tissue-engineered tissues cannot replace all skin functions. Protective barrier function is preserved, but touch and temperature sensation, perspiration, thermoregulation, protection from ultraviolet rays, and synthetic function are not restored [43,45], though several studies have investigated the possibility of re-establishing other skin functions with the combination of different cell types [46-48]. Skin-substitute products may be extracted from bone marrow cells [49], and the addition of skin appendages [50] or signaling molecules regulating cell-cell and cell-matrix interactions [51] has been studied to further functionalize bioconstructs.

Aesthetic results remain controversial. Issues of cosmesis and quality of life as well as functionality are nowadays to be considered altogether when dealing with skin-restoration treatment. Human skin does not regenerate postnatally; postnatal healing consists of repair rather than regeneration. Skin replacement products obtained from postnatal cellular materials are unlikely to obtain a true regeneration, and scarring is almost always the final consequence of the process [52,53]. As a matter of fact, skin repair results in scars formation. Uncontrolled scarring may cause possible loss of function where excessive tissue production and contraction occur, apart of poor aesthetic results. Hence, prevention of scar is a problem to be addressed after restoration of the damaged skin. Improved understanding of foetal wound healing has led to therapeutic measures directed at scar-free healing, mainly based on the principle that scarless healing is facilitated by a decreased inflammatory response [45,52]. It has been observed that during foetal life growth factors TGF-β1 and TGF-β2 are low or absent while TGF-β3 is higher; conversely, in adult individuals the latter is insignificant and TGF-β1 and –β2 are predominantly expressed during the inflammation phase of wound healing [54]. A complex interplay of these isoforms is crucial for optimal healing results, as studies on pig and human succeeded in reducing scarring by selectively increasing TGF-β3 and inhibiting TGF-β1 and -β2 levels, whilst neutralization of all three isoforms did not result in reduced scarring [54,55].

The role of stem cells has also been investigated. Both embryonic and adult stem cells have been used in several trials, but research on the former still is delayed by ethical debate. Adult stem cells are being used widely in different research fields. However, results are not as brilliant as expected, due to the impossibility of identifying a stem cell within human skin tissue without ambiguity [50,56,57] and also to unsuitable biochemical and mechanical conditions in a wound which may limit plasticity and proliferative activity of implanted stem cells [57]. Nevertheless, experimental studies conducted on murine models [50,58,59] suggest that research on stem cells should be encouraged as it may achieve production of fully functional true skin equivalents should pattern of cell differentiation be identified in human.

Author details

Silvestro Canonico*, Ferdinando Campitiello, Angela Della Corte, Vincenzo Padovano and Gianluca Pellino

*Address all correspondence to: silvestro.canonico@unina2.it

Department of Medical, Surgical, Neurologic, Metabolic and Ageing Sciences, Second University of Naples, Naples, Italy

References

[1] Schultz, G. S., & Wysocki, A. Interactions between extracellular matrix and growth factors in wound healing. Wound Repair Regen (2009). , 17(2), 153-62.

[2] Falanga, V. Classifications for wound bed preparation and stimulation of chronic wounds. Wound Repair Regen (2000). , 8, 347-52.

[3] Stanley, A., & Osler, T. Senescence and the healing rates of venous ulcers. J Vasc Surg (2001). , 33, 1206-11.

[4] Cook, H., Davies, K. J., Harding, K. G., & Thomas, D. W. Defective extracellular matrix reorganization by chronic wound fibroblasts is associated with alterations in TIMP-1, TIMP-2, and MMP-2 activity. J Invest Dermatol (2000). , 115, 225-33.

[5] Hasan, A., Murata, H., Falabella, A., et al. Dermal fibroblasts from venous ulcers are unresponsive to the action of transforming growth factor-beta 1. J Dermatol Sci (1997). , 16, 59-66.

[6] Agren, Steenfos. H. H., Dabelsteen, S., et al. Proliferation and mitogenic response to PDGF-BB of fibroblasts isolated from chronic venous leg ulcers is ulcer-age dependent. J Invest Dermatol (1999). , 112, 463-9.

[7] Mendez, M. V., Stanley, A., Park, H. Y., et al. Fibroblasts cultured from venous ulcers display cellular characteristics of senescence. J Vasc Surg (1998). , 28, 876-83.

[8] Van de Berg, J. S., Rudolph, R., Hollan, C., & Haywood-Reid, P. L. Fibroblast senescence in pressure ulcers. Wound Repair Regen (1998). , 6, 38-49.

[9] Gibson, D., Cullen, B., & Legerstee, R. (2009). Available from http://www.woundsinternational.com

[10] Frame, Still. J., Lakhel Le, Coadou. A., et al. Use of dermal regeneration template in contracture release procedures: a multicenter evaluation. Plast Reconstr Surg (2004). , 113, 1330-8.

[11] Mac, Neil. S. What role does the extracellular matrix serve in skin grafting and wound healing? Burns (1994). suppl 1): S, 67-70.

[12] Iwuagwu, F. C., Wilson, D., & Bailie, F. The use of skin grafts in postburn contracture release: a 10-year review. Plast Reconstr Surg (1999). , 103, 1198-207.

[13] Zhong SP, Zhang YZ, Lim CT.Tissue scaffolds for skin wound healing and dermal reconstruction. WIREs Nanomed Nanobiotechnol (2010). , 2, 510-25.

[14] International consensus.Acellular matrices for the treatment of wounds. An expert working group review. London: Wounds International, (2010).

[15] Matouskova, E., Broz, L., Sotbova, et al. Human allogeneic keratinocytes cultured on acellular xenodermis: the use in healing of burns and other skin defects. Biomed Mater Eng (2006). suppl 4): SS71., 63.

[16] Brychta, P., Adler, J., Rihova, H., et al. Cell Tissue Bank (2002). , 3, 15-23.

[17] Erdag, G., & Morgan, J. R. Allogeneic versus xenogeneic immune reaction to bioengineered skin grafts. Cell Transplant (2004). , 13, 701-12.

[18] Nataraj, C., Ritter, G., Dumas, S., et al. Wounds (2007). , 19(6), 148-56.

[19] Morimoto, N., Saso, Y., Tomihata, K., et al. Viability and function of autologous and allogeneic fibroblasts seeded in dermal substitutes after implantation. J Surg Res (2005). , 125, 56-67.

[20] Dantzer, E., Queruel, P., Salinier, L., et al. Dermal regeneration template for deep hand burns: clinical utility for both eatly grafting and reconstructive surgery. Br J Plast Surg (2003). , 56, 764-74.

[21] Rennekampff, H. O., Hansbrough, J. F., Woods, V., & Jr Kiessig, V. Integrin and matrix molecule expression in cultured skin replacements. J Burn Care Rehabil (1996). , 17, 213-21.

[22] Griffiths, M., Ojeh, N., Livingstone, R., et al. Survival of Apligraf in acute human wounds. Tissue Eng (2004). , 10, 1180-95.

[23] Cullen, B., Watt, P. W., Lundqvist, C., et al. The role of oxidised regenerated cellulose/collagen in chronic wound repair and its potential mechanism of action. Int J Biochem Cell Biol (2002). , 34(12), 1544-56.

[24] Brown-Etris, M., Cutshall, W. D., & Hiles, M. C. Wounds (2002). , 50-66.

[25] Voytik-Harbin SL, Brightman AO, Kraine MR, et al.Identification of extractable growth factors from small intestine submucosa. J Cell Biochem (1997). , 57, 478-91.

[26] Hodde JP, Record RD, Liang HA, Badylak SF.Vascular endothelial growth factor in porcinederived extracellular matrix. Endothelium (2001). , 8(1), 11-24.

[27] Cornwell, K. G., Landsman, A., & James, K. S. Extracellular matrix biomaterials for soft tissue repair. Clin Podiatr Med Surg (2009). , 26, 507-23.

[28] Powell HM, Boyce ST. EDC cross-linking improves skin substitute strength and stability. (2006). *Biomaterials*, 27(34), 5821-27.

[29] Wiegland, C., Abel, M., Ruth, P., & Hipler, U. C. Influence of the collagen origin on the binding affinity for neutrophil elastase. Abstract presented at: 18th Conference of the European Wound Management Association (EWMA); May (2008)., 14-16.

[30] Mulder, G., & Lee, D. K. Wounds (2009)., 21(9), 254-61.

[31] 2003, Sheehan, P., Jones, P., Caselli, A., et al. Percent change in wound area of diabetic foot ulcers over a 4-week period is a robust predictor of complete healing in a 12-week prospective trial. *Diabetes Care*, 26(6), 1879-82.

[32] Burke JF, Yannas IV, Quinby WC Jr, et al.Successful use of a physiologically acceptable artificial skin in the treatment of extensive burn injury. Ann Surg (1981). , 194, 413-20.

[33] Dostal GH, Gamelli RL. Fetal wound healing.Surg Gynecol Obstet (1993). , 176, 299-306.

[34] Bullard, K. M., Longaker, M. T., & Lorenz, H. P. (2003). 27, 54-61.

[35] Olutoye OO, Barone EJ, Yager DR.Hyaluronic acid inhibits fetal platelet function: implications in scarless healing. J Pediatr Surg (1997)., 32, 1037-40.

[36] Gottlieb, Furman. J. Successful management and surgical closure of chronic and pathological wounds using Integras. J Burns Surg Wound Care (2004)., 3, 54-60.

[37] Moiemen NS, Staiano JJ, Ojeh NO, et al.Reconstructive surgery with a dermal regeneration template: clinical and histologic study. Plast Reconstr Surg (2001). , 108, 93-103.

[38] Orgill DP, Straus FH II, Lee RC.The use of collagen-GAG membranes in reconstructive surgery. Ann NY Acad Sci (1999)., 888, 233-48.

[39] Heimbach, D., Luterman, A., Burke, J., et al. Artificial dermis for major burns: a multi-center randomized clinical trial. Ann Surg (1988)., 208, 313-20.

[40] Sheridan, R. L., Hegarty, M., Tompkins, R. G., et al. Artificial skin in massive burns: results to ten years. Eur J Plast Surg (1994)., 17, 91-3.

[41] Heimbach, D. M., Warden, G. D., Luterman, A., et al. Multicenter postapproval clinical trial of Integra dermal regeneration template for burn treatment. J Burn Care Rehabil (2003)., 24, 42-8.

[42] Chou TD, Chen SL, Lee TW, et al.Reconstruction of burn scar of the upper extremities with artificial skin. Plast Reconstr Surg (2001)., 108, 378-84.

[43] Mac, Neil. S. (2007). Progress and opportunities for tissue-engineered skin. *Nature*, 445, 874-80.

[44] Boyce ST, Kagan RJ, Greenhalgh DG, et al.Cultured skins substitutes reduce requirements for harvesting of skin autograft for closure of excised, full-thickness burns. J Trauma (2006)., 60, 821-9.

[45] Metcalfe AD, Ferguson MW.Tissue engineering of replacement skin: the crossroads of biomaterials, wound healing, embryonic development, stem cells and regeneration. J R Soc Interface (2007). , 4, 413-37.

[46] Ponec, M., El Ghalbzouri, A., Dijkman, R., et al. (2004). Endothelial network formed with human dermal microvascular endothelial cells in autologous multicellular skin substitutes. *Angiogenesis*, 7, 295-305.

[47] Dezutter-Dambuyant, C., Black, A., Bechetoille, N., et al. Biomed Mater Eng (2006). S, 85-94.

[48] Rolin, G., Placet, V., Jacquet, E., et al. Development and characterization of a human dermal equivalent with physiological mechanical properties. Skin Res Technol (2012). , 18, 251-8.

[49] Fioretti, F., Lebreton-Decoster, C., Gueniche, F., et al. Human bone-marrow derived cells: an attractive source to populate dermal substitutes. Wound Repair Regen (2008). , 16, 87-94.

[50] Blanpain, C., Lowry, W. E., Geoghegan, A., et al. Cell (2004). , 118, 635-48.

[51] Ma PX.Biomimetic materials for tissue engineering. Adv Drug Deliv Rev (2008). , 60, 184-98.

[52] Martin, P., & Leibowich, S. J. Inflammatory cells during wound repair: the good, the bad and the ugly. Trend Cell Biol (2005). , 15, 599-607.

[53] Metcalfe AD, Ferguson MW. (2007). Bioengineering skin using mechanisms of regeneration and repair. *Biomaterials*, 28, 5100-13.

[54] Ferguson, M. W., & O'Kane, S. Phil Trans R Soc Lond B (2004). , 359, 839-50.

[55] O'Kane, S., & Ferguson, M. W. Transforming growth factor βs and wound healing. Int J Biochem Cell Biol (1997). , 29, 63-78.

[56] Tumbar, T. Epithelial skin stem cells. Methods Enzymol (2006). , 419, 73-99.

[57] Lemoli, R. M., Bertolini, F., Cancedda, R., et al. (2005). 90, 360-81.

[58] Toma, J. G., Akhavan, M., Fernandes, K. J., et al. Isolation of multipotent adult stem cells from the dermis of mammalian skin. Nat Cell Biol (2001). , 3, 778-84.

[59] Blanpain, C., Horsley, V., & Fuchs, E. Cell (2007). , 128, 445-58.

Chapter 6

Useful Tips for Skin Grafts

Rei Ogawa and Hiko Hyakusoku

Additional information is available at the end of the chapter

http://dx.doi.org/10.5772/55084

1. Introduction

Skin grafting is a common operative procedure that is widely used in plastic, reconstructive, and aesthetic surgery. Beyond mere graft survival, however, the goals of surgery include good matching of texture and color and minimizing donor morbidity. These factors and optimal donor sites require careful consideration in each patient. We have found that the recommendations offered below can help achieve these goals.

2. Skin-graft harvesting on the basis of a high-cut bathing suit

When harvesting full-thickness skin grafts, it is important to consider each patient's age and sex to select the appropriate donor sites [1]. The correct color and texture is of paramount importance, but also important is minimal donor-site morbidity. The favored donor sites usually include the postauricular and subclavicular regions, the medial side of the upper arm, and the inguinal region. Of these sites, the inguinal region is often preferred because of its inconspicuous position and the facility of primary closure (Fig1a, b). However, a wound on the crease of inguinal region is much more objectionable than we had expected, especially for young female patients, because of the current vogue for swimsuits and short pants with high-cut leg openings. An example of such a case is that of a young woman in whom we selected the inguinal region as the donor site. Moreover, the crease of the inguinal region is often pigmented because of chronic inflammation due to sweat or sebum. It is, therefore, best to focus on the high-cut leg region rather than the inguinal crease (Fig1c, d). Another benefit of this approach is that the patient can be permitted to walk immediately after the operation, because when the legs are moved a wound in the high-cut leg region is subjected to less tension than is a wound in the inguinal region. This method should be indicated in female infant patients for the future.

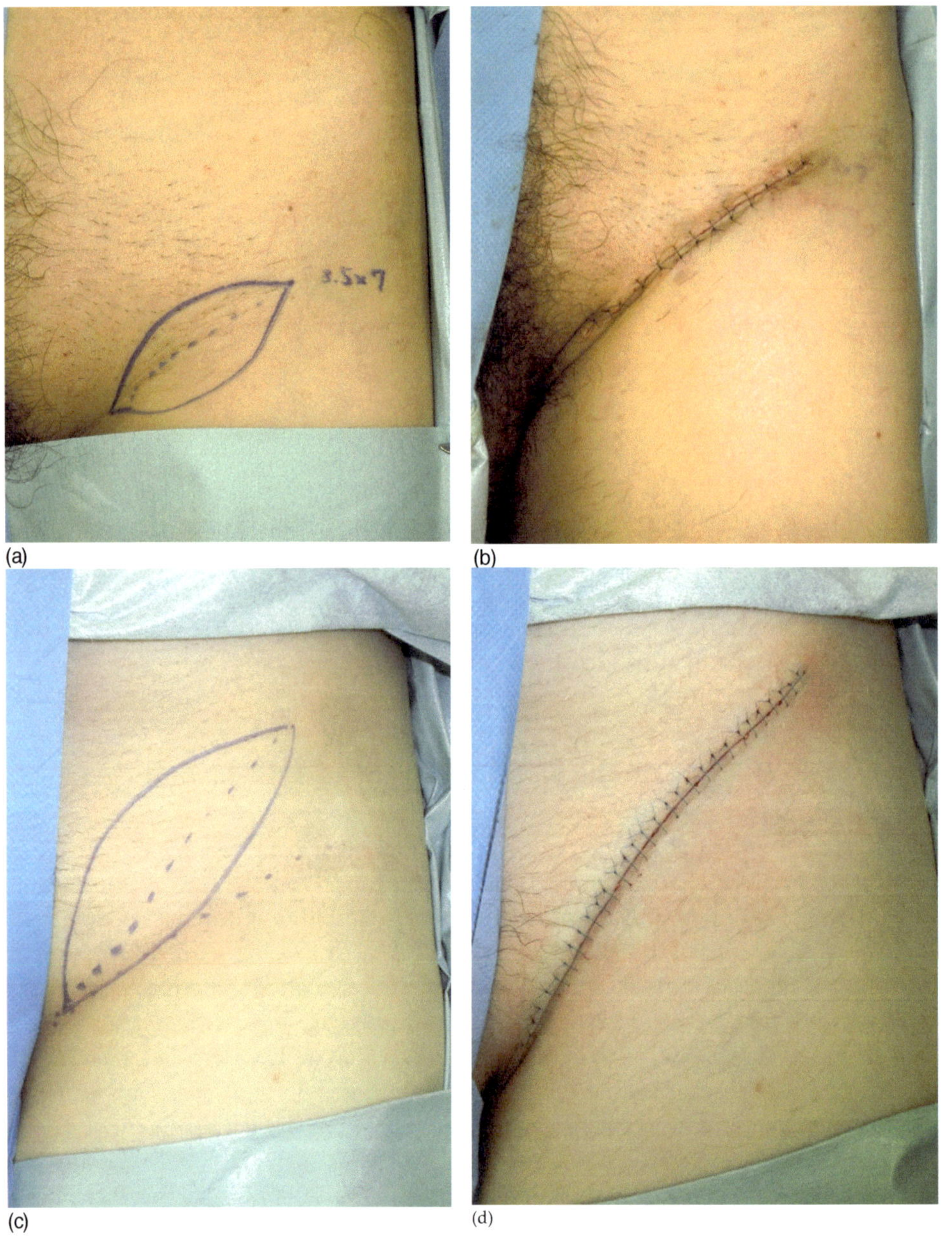

Figure 1. (a) Design of harvesting a skin graft on the conventional inguinal region (b) The sutured wound on the inguinal crease (c) Design of harvesting a skin graft on the our on the high-cut leg region (d) The sutured wound on the high-cut leg region

http://dx.doi.org/10.5772/55084

3. Use of a flower holder for making drainage holes

The success of a skin graft depends on [1] appropriate debridement of the recipient site down to the layer providing the blood supply; [2] adequate hemostasis of the recipient site to prevent the development of a hematoma; and [3] sufficient compression and securing of skin grafts from corner to corner, using a tie-over dressing or bandages. Hemostasis is especially important in blood-rich regions such as the scalp, face, and hand. In such cases, drainage holes — which are also useful for the drainage of bacteria and exudates — should be made on the skin grafts. However, large drainage holes will leave scars; therefore, numerous small holes are preferred. To make such holes, a Japanese *kenzan* flower holder (Fig. 2a) is far more effective than surgical knives or needles. The graft, held by a rubber sheet, is turned onto a flower holder. It is then beaten (against the rubber sheet) with a hammer (Fig.2b). In this way, numerous small holes can be made in a matter of minutes (Fig. 2c). These holes suffice for drainage and become epithelialized after about 10 days (Fig. 2d, e). When using a flower holder for making drainage holes, split-thickness skin grafting is a good indication. When harvesting split-thickness skin grafts, it is important to select the non-outstanding donor sites..The favored donor sites usually include the thigh, the abdomen, and the dorsal region.

One established drainage method involves creating holes in the graft, typically with a No. 11 surgical knife. However, such holes can cause scars, so this method is undesirable when skin grafting is performed in exposed areas such as the face and dorsum of the hand. Before developing the method described here, we had used to create holes using an 18-gauge injection needle. However, uniformly creating numerous small holes took considerable time with large skin grafts. Non-expanded mesh skin grafts are also an option for treating actively bleeding wounds, but they are of limited use for cosmetic purposes.

4. Use of a tie-over dressing with external wire-frame fixation

We have used external wire-frame fixation for skin grafts since 1986. In 1991, we reported this method and described two advantages: [1] the technique is useful for securing grafts to wound beds and [2] preventing the graft edges from lifting [2]. Moreover, we confirmed the usefulness of this technique for skin grafting to regions with free borders, such as the lips and eyelids [3]. Particularly for eyelid grafts, external wire-frame fixation overcomes the disadvantages of tarsorrhaphy [3]. Moreover, this method can also be used for digital skin grafting [4]. Three-dimensional external wire frames are useful for fixing digital joints as well as skin grafts. If this method is used for digital skin grafts, the fixing of digital joints by pinning is not necessary, particularly for grafting the palmar surface of a finger.

During surgery, the skin graft is fixed with sutures by the usual method. At the same time, the wire frame, shaped like the graft itself, is made of 1.2-mm-diameter Kirschner wire. Then, one part of each suture is bound up (Fig. 3a, b), and the wire frame is applied to the graft. Next, the wire frame is attached with the same sutures already used for stitching the graft. Finally, tie-over fixation is performed in the usual way (Fig.3c). The skin graft is then taken from corner to corner even if it involves application on a free edge. This method is helpful to secure the skin graft after operation, and the post operative course will be uneventful (Fig.3d).

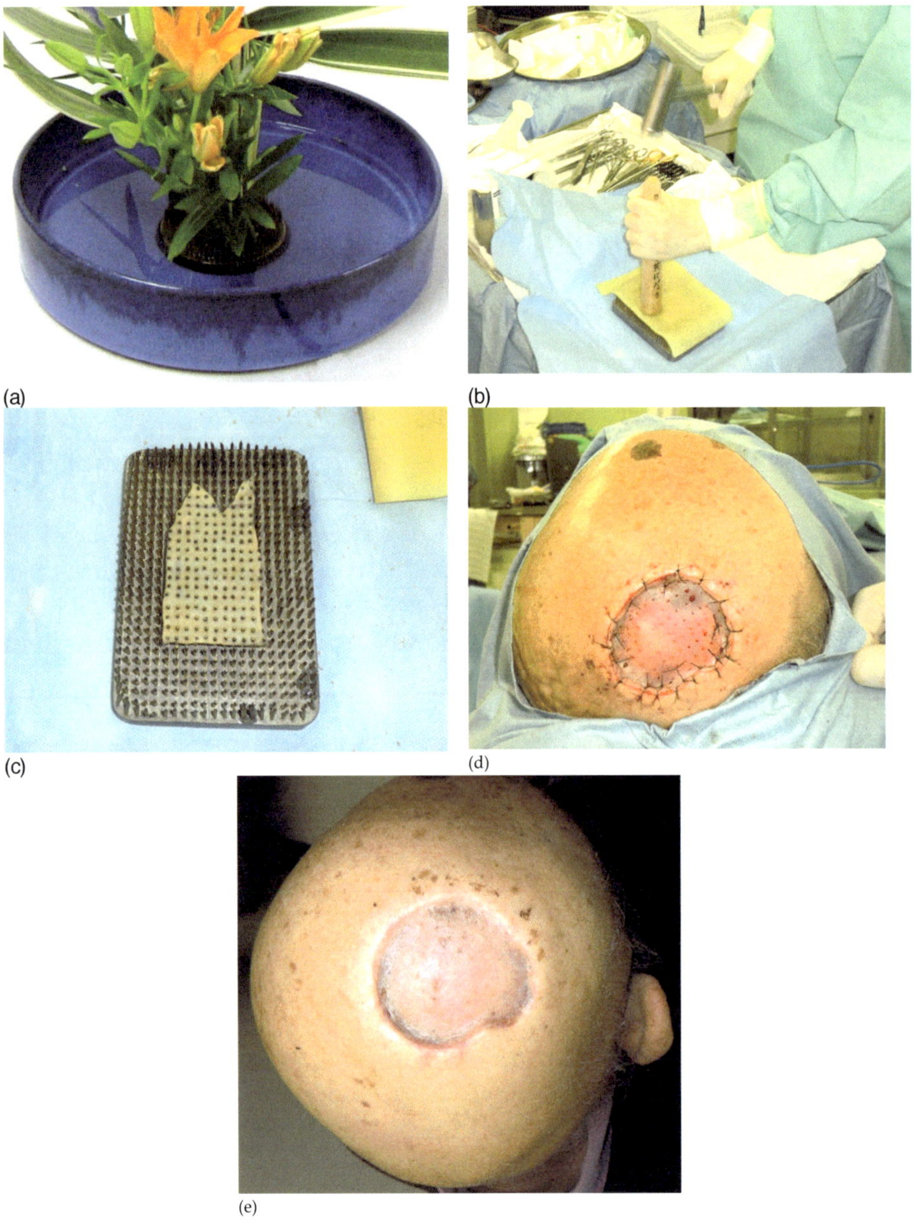

Figure 2. (a) A Japanese Kenzan flower holder (b) Making holes by beaten with a hammer (c) Numerous small holes (d) Immediately after skin grafting: blood is drainaged from holes (e) A month after operation: there are no scars of drainage holes

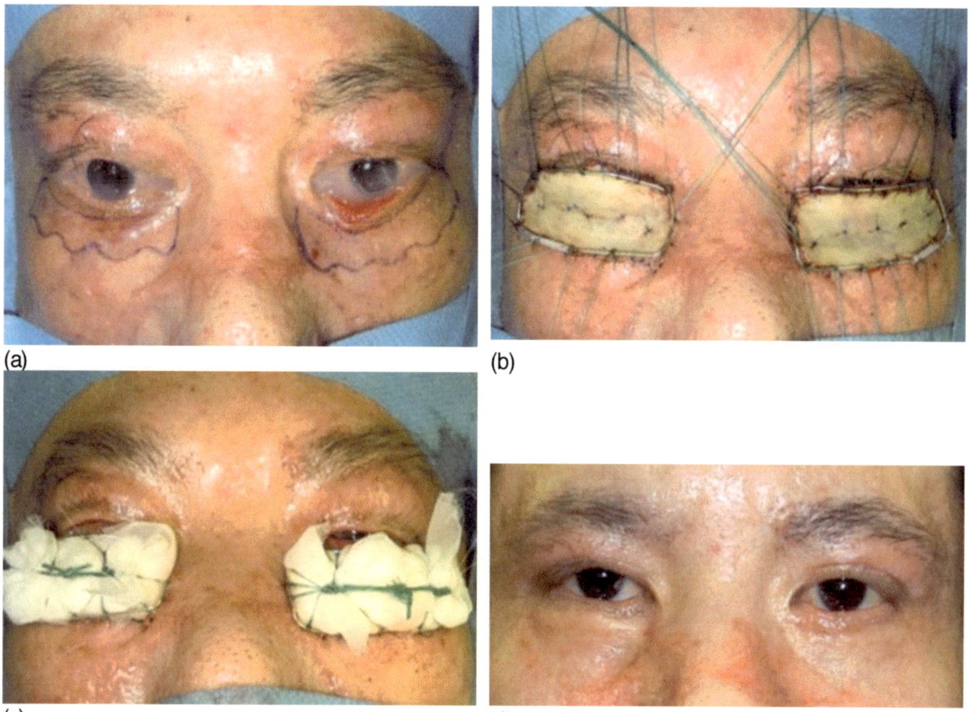

(a) (b) (c) (d)

Figure 3. (a) Preoperative view of scar contractures on the bilateral lower eyelids (b) After applying skin grafts and external wire frames (c) Tie-over fixation (d) 6 months post operative view: scar contracture is completely released

5. Conclusions

We have presented three techniques that we have found to reduce complications and surgical invasiveness. [1] Skin grafts should be harvested on the basis of a swimsuit with high-cut leg openings. [2] A flower holder is recommended for making drainage holes. [3] A tie-over dressing using external wire-frame fixation is recommended. As mentioned, the success of a skin graft depends on: [1] appropriate debridement of the recipient site down to the layer providing the blood supply; [2] adequate hemostasis of the recipient site to prevent the development of a hematoma; and [3] sufficient compression and securing of skin grafts from corner to corner, using a tie-over dressing or bandages. However, most important is the surgeon's determination to reduce complications and surgical invasiveness. With this attitude, we have developed these recommendations. We hope that they will become widely known among the many physicians working with patients who require surgery of this kind.

Author details

Rei Ogawa and Hiko Hyakusoku

*Address all correspondence to: r.ogawa@nms.ac.jp

Department of Plastic, Reconstructive and Aesthetic Surgery, Nippon Medical School, Tokyo, Japan

References

[1] Rigg, B. M. Importance of donor site selection in skin grafting. Can Med Assoc J (1977). , 117, 1028-29.

[2] Hirai, T, Hyakusoku, H, & Fumiiri, M. The use of a wire frame to fix grafts externally. Br J Plast Surg (1991). , 44, 69-70.

[3] Murakami, M, Hyakusoku, H, & Ishimaru, S. External wire frame fixation of eyelid graft. Br J Plast Surg (2003). , 56, 312-13.

[4] Ogawa, R, Aoki, S, Aoki, M, Oki, K, & Hyakusoku, H. Three-dimensional external skin graft fixation of digital skin graft. Plast Reconstr Surg (2007). IN PRESS.

Section 3

Management of Donor Area

Chapter 7

Polyethylene Surgical Drape Dressing for Split Thickness Skin Graft Donor Areas

Madhuri A. Gore, Kabeer Umakumar and Sandhya P. Iyer

Additional information is available at the end of the chapter

http://dx.doi.org/10.5772/54195

1. Introduction

A variety of dressings has been used for covering the split thickness skin graft donor areas. Some of these are alginates, collagen sheets, films and the most commonly used impregnated tulle gras dressing. The chief goal of management of donor area is to achieve early epithelisation without infection. Minimum pain, easy availability and low cost of dressing are other desirable criteria. A controlled clinical trial was conducted to compare Vaseline impregnated gauze and Banana leaf dressing (BLD) (Fig 1) developed at the burn unit at LTM medical college and hospital in 1997. [1] The results showed BLD to be effective with significantly less pain and at much lower cost.

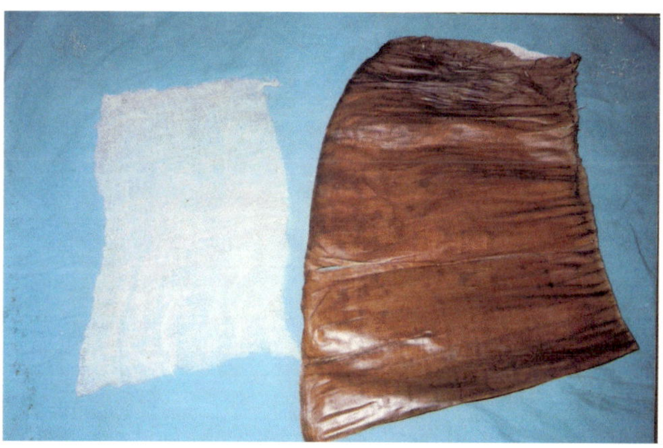

Figure 1. Vaseline impregnated gauze and autoclaved banana leaf dressing

While BLD needs to be prepared, polyethylene surgical drape (PSD) (Fig 2) is readily available. Hence it was decided to compare the efficacy of PSD with already established BLD as dressing for skin graft donor areas.

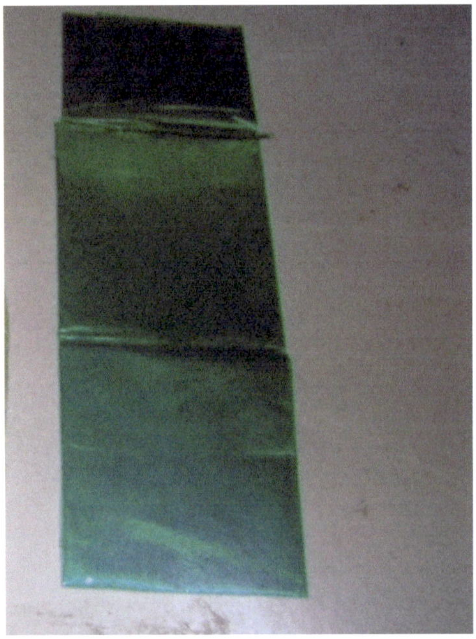

Figure 2. Polyethylene surgical drape

2. Materials and methods

A prospective controlled study was conducted in fifty patients of either sex between 18 to 65 years of age undergoing split thickness skin grafting - STSG. The patients were blinded to the type of dressing applied on the donor area till the first dressing change. The study protocol was approved by the Institutional Ethics Committee prior to commencement of the study. Informed written consent was obtained from every patient prior to enrollment in the study.

3. Patient inclusion criteria

- Patients between 18 to 65 years of age
- Patients of either sex
- Patients undergoing STSG with thigh as donor area

- Surgery under general anaesthesia

4. Patient exclusion criteria

- Patients with diabetes or hypertension
- Pregnant females
- Patients in whom area other than thigh was used as donor site.
- Surgery under regional anaesthesia.

5. Banana leaf dressing preparation

Banana leaf dressing was prepared by cutting the midrib of the leaf and then pasting the leaf on a piece of bandage cloth with thin paste made by cooking fine flour. These dressings were then hung on clothes' drying stand for 24 hours for the paste to dry. The dressing was rolled; packed in paper bag and autoclaved and was then ready for use.

6. Polyethylene surgical drape dressing

A single sheet of ethylene oxide sterlised polyethylene surgical drape available at the hospital was used in this study. It was cut appropriately to match the size of the donor area.

7. Trial protocol

Split thickness skin grafts were harvested from one or both thighs using Humby's skin grafting handle fitted with number 12 skin grafting blade. Partial thickness of donor areas was judged by the appearance of punctate hemorrhages. Gauze pieces soaked in adrenaline: saline (1:300,000) solution were applied over the raw surface to achieve haemostasis over donor areas.

After ensuring haemostasis the upper half of donor area (Area A - control) was dressed with BLD while the lower half was dressed with PSD dressing (Area B - study) (Fig 3). Both the dressings were covered with gamjee pad rolls and then firmly bandaged.

All patients were blinded to the type of dressing applied over a given area as the dressing was applied while the patients were under of general anesthesia. The patient remained blinded till the first dressing change.

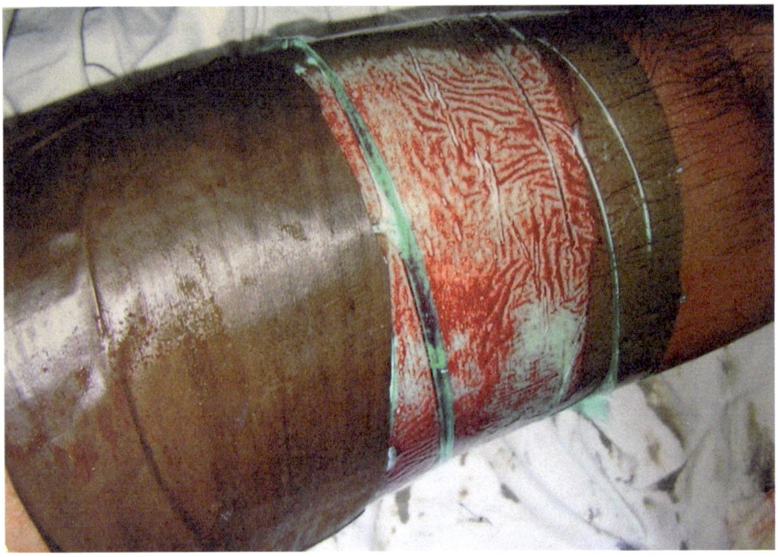

Figure 3. Application of BLD and PSD on donor area

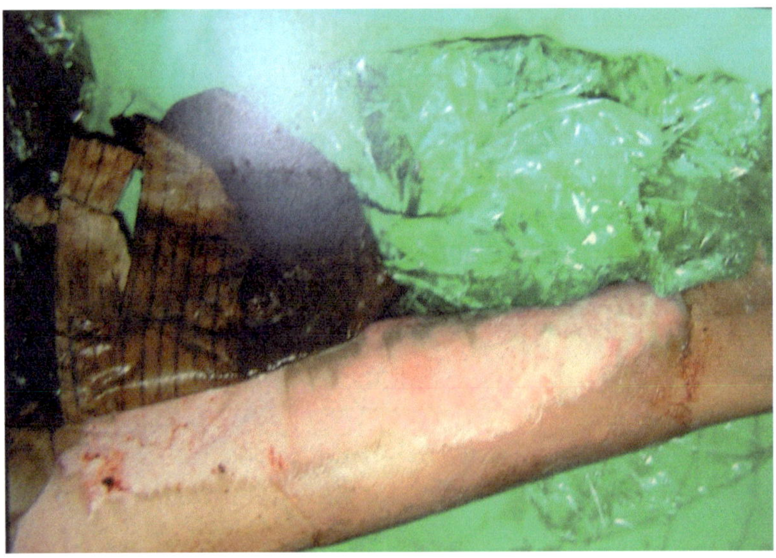

Figure 4. Epithelisation under BLD and PSD

The dressing on donor area was opened on 7th post-harvest day, unless indicated earlier. Thereafter, the dressing was changed and area was inspected every day till complete epithelisation. (Fig 4)

8. The following observations were made

1. Age and sex of patient
2. Status of donor area epithelisation on seventh post-harvest day.
3. Evidence of donor area infection
4. Days needed for complete epithelisation
5. Background and dressing removal pain scores.

9. The following scores were evaluated

1. Background pain score : The patients were asked to award a score from 0 to 10 on visual analogue scale for each of the areas under the two different dressing materials on day 1 and day 3 post harvest (before they underwent first dressing change)
2. Dressing removal pain score : The patients were asked to award a score from 0 to 10 for each of the dressing materials while the dressing was being removed on 7th day post harvest and at subsequent dressing changes.

The data obtained; was analysed and subjected to test of statistical significance using paired 't' test.

10. Results

From Jan 2009 to July 2009, 50 patients undergoing STSG were included in this study. The patient population included significantly more number of females younger than 33 years of age. The average age of males and females in our study was 41.54 and 27.63 years, respectively. This difference was statistically highly significant (P=0.000) (Table 1)

Age group in yrs	Sex				Total
	Male		Female		
18-33	11	42.3%	19	79.2%	30(60%)
34-49	5	19.2%	5	20.8%	10(20%)
50-65	10	38.5%	0	0%	10(20%)
Total	26	100%	24	100%	50(100%)

Table 1. Age and sex distribution of patients in both the groups

Average donor area covered under each dressing material was 177cm^2

(Range : Minimum area – 156 sq cm; maximum area – 198 sq cm)

Complete epithelisation of donor area was seen in 37 patients (74%) on 7th post-harvest day in both study and control group. Out of the thirteen patients with incomplete epithelisation on 7th post-harvest day under both BLD & PSD; 11 donor areas under BLD and 12 donor areas under PSD dressing were completely epithelised on 9th post-harvest day. So, a total of 48 donor areas (96%) under BLD and 49 donor areas (98%) under PSD dressing epithelised completely by 9th post-harvest day. The remaining 3 donor areas showed complete epitheli-sation by day 11 post harvest. There was no evidence of infection of donor areas under both BLD and PSD dressing in this study (Table 2)

Post harvest days	**Status of epithilisation**	**Groups of Areas**	
		A (Control)	**B(Study)**
Day 7 post-harvest	Complete	37(74%)	37(74%)
	Incomplete	13(28%)	13(26%)
Day 9 post-harvest	Complete	48(96%)	49(98%)
	Incomplete	02(4%)	01(2%)
Infection		0	0

A : Group of areas under BLD B : Group of areas under PSD

Table 2. Status of epithalisation of donor areas on day 7 and day 9 post-harvest

The average time taken for complete epithelisation of donor area under BLD was 7.6 ± 1.087 days and it was 7.56 ± 0.993 days under PSD. This difference was not significant statistically (P=0.322) (Table 3)

Time taken in days for complete epithelisation		**Groups of Areas**	
		A(Control)	**B(Study)**
Mean number of days taken	X ± SD	7.6 ± 1.087	7.56 ± 0.993
Range in days taken for complete epithelisation	Minimum	7	7
	Maximum	11	11

A : Group of areas under BLD B : Group of areas under PSD

Table 3. Time taken for complete epithelisation

The background pain scores under PSD dressing were significantly less than that under BLD on day 1 and day 3 post-harvest (day 1, P = 0.002 & day 3; p= 0.000). There was also

http://dx.doi.org/10.5772/54195

highly significant decrease in background pain scores on day 3 post -harvest under both BLD & PSD dressing. This mean decrease in background pain under BLD from day 1 to day 3 was 1.48 (p=0.000) while the same under PSD dressing was 1.64 (p=0.000). This difference in mean decrease was not statistically significant (Table 4)

Days post harvest	Background pain scores		Groups of Areas	
			A(Control)	B(Study)
Day 1	Range	Minimum	3	2
		Maximum	6	6
	Mean	(X ± SD)	4.82 ± 0.941	4.52 ± 1.035
Day 3	Range	Minimum	2	2
		Maximum	5	5
	Mean	(X ± SD)	3.34 ± 0.823*	2.88 ± 0.824**

Decrease in background pain score * Group A (P = 0.000) **Group B (P=0.000) Highly significant

Table 4. Background pain score on day 1 (d1) & day 3 (d3) post-harvest.

The dressing removal pain scores under PSD dressing were significantly less than that under BLD on both the days i.e. day 7 and day 9 post-harvest. There was a decrease in dressing removal pain scores on day 9 post-harvest under both BLD and PSD dressings. This mean decrease under PSD dressing was (0.583 ± 0.660) statistically significant while the same under BLD was (0.076 + 0.76) not statistically significant. The difference in mean decrease in pain scores in both the groups was 0.461 which though not significant (p=0.082) was close to significance (Table 5)

Days post harvest	Dressing Removal pain scores		Groups of Areas	
			A(Control)	B(Study)
Day 7	Range	Minimum	6	1
		Maximum	9	4
	Mean	(X ± SD)	8.42 + 0.731	2.34 ± 0.658*
Day 9	Range	Minimum	6	1
		Maximum	9	3
	Mean	(X ± SD)	8.384± 0.870	2.00 ± 0.408**

Difference in dressing removal pain scores in group (A & B) on day 7 * (P=0.000) and day 9 ** (P=0.000) Highly significant

Table 5. Dressing removal pain score on day 7 (d7) & day 9 (d9) post-harvest

The cost of 100cm^2 of BLD is 20 paise while that of 100cm^2 of PSD is 26.19 paise. Both these dressing materials are very cheap especially when compared to commercially available paraffin impregnated gauze dressing (Rupees 5.80 per 100cm^2) and collagen dressing (Rupees 175 per 100cm^2) (Table 6) (1 Rupee = 100 paise, 1 $ == 54 Rs)

Sr. no.	Material	Average cost in Rupees per 100 cm^2
1	Collagen	175
2	Vaseline/ Paraffin Impregnated gauze	5.80
3	PSD	0.262
4	BLD	0.20

Rs 1 = 100 paise, $ 1 = 54 Rs

Table 6. Cost comparison of donor site dressing materials

11. Discussion

Every year about 7-8 million people suffer from burn injury in India and approximately 0.2 million die. [2] At our burns unit in Mumbai, we treat about 600 patients with burns every year and this accounts for 1.5% of total hospital admissions. Our own data shows that the average per capita monthly income of the patients admitted in our unit is less than Rs. 200. This is true for majority of burns victims in India.[1]

Skin grafting is an integral component of burn management for achieving wound closure in full thickness burn wounds[3]. The need for early epithelisation of STSG donor area in burn patients cannot be overemphasized as donor sites may be limited and reharvesting may be needed to obtain wound closure.

The pain experienced by the patients in the postoperative period is more at the donor area than at the recipient site. It may make the patients reluctant to undergo further procedures. [4] Till date, there is no consensus regarding the optimal donor site dressing that would result in early healing with minimal or no pain at the donor area. [5],[6],[7] Petroleum Jelly impregnated gauze i.e. Vaseline gauze (VG) is the most commonly used dressing for STSG donor areas in majority of centers. But in a study conducted at our Burns unit in the past, we observed that this dressing was not completely non adherent and the pain experienced by the patients was signficiant.[1]

The ideal dressing for STSG donor area should be painless when applied, non- adherent, non – toxic, non – antigenic, cheap, easily available and should achieve epithelisation of the STSG donor areas as early as possible. Non- adhesive dressings are ideal for these areas as they are not only pain free but also minimize damage to the new epidermis during dressing removal thus aiding the process of healing. A study conducted in 1996-97 comparing BLD with VG, proved that BLD is a more suitable dressing for STSG donor areas and also, the cheapest of all the available dressings.[1]

Polythelene surgical drape is made up of polythelene which is an artificial inert chemical compound impermeable to gases and water. It has a smooth surface which allows it to fall off when the outer dressing is removed. It is very commonly used at our center as an integral part of surgical draping before carrying out any surgical procedure. So it is easily available in the hospital as ethylene oxide sterilized, ready to use packs and is provided free of cost to the patients from the hospital supply. Commercially available polyethelne surgical drape costs 26.19 paise per $100cm^2$. (Rs 55 for sheet size 140 X 150 cm). So, we decided to evaluate the efficacy of PSD as STSG donor site dressing and compare it with BLD which is the most commonly used dressing material for STSG donor areas at our center.

The review of literature failed to reveal any reference about the use of PSD as a dressing material. However, various researchers have tried out many different materials in an effort to identify the most ideal STSG donor site dressing.

Persson K and Salemark L found that polyurethane film caused less pain and discomfort and was also the easiest to remove amongst paraffin gauze, polyurethane foam, polyethane film and polyurethane film. [8] Similar findings were observed by Weber RS et al in the trial comparing polyurethane foam dressing with a petroleum gauze dressing. [9] Lawrence J E and Blake GB compared scarlet red with calcium alginate as a dressing material for STSG donor sites [10] Misir liogly A et al have used honey for STSG donor sites [11] Yadav JK et al in their study compared topical phenytoin with conventional antibiotic impregnated tulle dressing (Sofratulle) and polyurethane membrane drape (Opsite) [12]. Santamaria AB et al have tried out hydrocolloid dressings [13] and P Halankar et al have tested collagen sheets in their study [14]. But none of these studies have been able to establish the superiority of one dressing over the other and question of ideal STSG donor site dressing remains unanswered.

Fifty patients of either sex and between 18 to 65 years of age undergoing STSG were included in our study. As the dressings were applied in the operating theatre while the patient was under general anaesthesia, the patient was blinded to the type of dressing till the first dressing change.

The study subjects included significantly higher number of young females. This corresponds with the generally higher incidence of burn injury in young females as compared to males.

Epithellisation was complete in 37 donor areas (74%) under BLD (control) as well as PSD(study) dressing on the seventh post-harvest day. In addition, 11 (22%) donor areas under BLD and 12 (24%) donor areas under PSD dressing epithelised completely on the ninth post -harvest day. So, ninety six percent donor areas (48) under BLD and 98%(49) donor areas under PSD dressing had healed completely by ninth post-harvest day. The average number of days required for complete epithelisation under BLD and PSD dressing were similar, that is 7.6 ± 1.087 and 7.57 ± 0.993 days, respectively. Gore reported significantly earlier healing with BLD as compared to VG dressing (8.67 days with BLD and 11.73 days with VG dressing) [1]. Horch RE and Stark GB found complete donor site healing within 7.5 days with collagen dressing and 12.5 days with polyurethane film dressing [15]. In another Indian study by Yadav JK and Singhvi AM, mean time for complete healing of donor areas under topical phenytoin, opsite and tulle dressings was 6.2, 8.6 and 12.6 days, respectively [12] Our study shows that PSD dressing is as effective as BLD as a STSG donor site dressing material in achieving complete epithelisation in shorter time period than tulle dressings and polyurethane film dressing.

The background pain score was significantly less for donor areas covered by PSD dressing than those covered by BLD The mean background pain score decreased significantly on day 3 post-harvest (3.34 for BLD & 2.88 for PSD dressing) from day 1 post-harvest (4.82 for BLD and 4.52 for PSD dressing) for both BLD and PSD dressing.

Thirteen patients (26%) in both the groups required second dressing change on day 9 as their donor sites had not completely epithelised by day 7. The mean dressing removal pain score was significantly less (2.34 on day 7 and 2.00 on day 9 post-harvest)for PSD covered areas than those covered with BLD (8.42 on day 7 and 8.38 on day 9 post-harvest). The difference in dressing removal pain scores between the groups (A & B) was highly significant on day 7 (P=0.000) as well as day 9 (P=0.000).So PSD dressing covered donor areas had significantly less pain and discomfort as compared to BLD covered donor areas.

Gore had observed BLD offered better pain relief and led to earlier epithelisation as compared to VG dressing.1 So, it is apparent that both PSD dressing and BLD are far superior to VG dressing in terms of STSG donor site pain as well as donor site healing. Hence, their use is recommended over VG for dressing of STSG donor areas.

Today the cost of banana leaf dressing is 20 paise per 100cm^2 (Rs 3.00 for dressing size 75 cms X 20 cms) and it is 26.19 paise per 100 cm^2 for PSD dressing (Rs 55.00 for sheet size 140 cms x 150 cms). So both these dressing materials are much cheaper than collagen dressing which is the most expensive with a cost of Rs. 175 per 100 cm^2 (Kollagen; company Eucare). Even the cheapest of vaseline / paraffin impregnated gauze dressing which is used in many other centers costs RS. 5.80 per 100cm$^{2.}$ (Rs 58 for 10 sheets of 10 x 10 cm –Jelonet) Many burnt patients need use of large donor areas. So the actual cost of these expensive donor site dressings is prohibitive for majority of burn victims in India. Hence both BLD which is the cheapest and PSD dressing which is also very cheap, are effective and economical donor site dressing materials with shorter healing time and lesser pain.

There was no evidence of donor area infection under BLD as well as PSD dressing in our study. There were no local as well as systemic allergic reactions observed while using PSD. However, soakage of the secondary dressing was found in a significantly higher number of donor areas (32 i.e. 64%) covered by BLD than those covered by PSD dressing (21 i.e. 42%). This may be due to the fact that during preparation, rolling and autoclaving process, BLD develops a few cracks. These cracks allow the egress of exudate. This can be taken care by providing extra layers of gamjee pads. However, it did not warrant earlier dressing change.

Twenty one (42%) PSD covered donor areas showed soakage with seepage of yellowish exudate. This may be due to the fact that PSD is an artificial membrane which does not absorb wound exudates at all. This exudate then seeps under the dressing and also soaks the outer layers. This can be tackled by making slits in PSD before it is applied so that, exudate can come out through these slits and get absorbed in the secondary dressing of gamjee pad.. Even though, PSD literally falls off the donor site once the outer supporting layer is removed during dressing change, there was not a single case of slippage of dressing in PSD covered donor areas.

12. Conclusions

1. Polyethelene surgical drape is as effective as Banana leaf dressing for STSG donor area dressing.
2. Polyethelene surgical drape caused less background pain as well as dressing change pain as compared to banana leaf dressing.
3. Polyethelene surgical drape though little more expensive than Banana leaf dressing, is cheaper than all the other conventional dressings.

Thus, polyethylene surgical drape is a non-adherent, non-allergic, non- antigenic, cheap, easily available, effective and acceptable alternative dressing for split thickness skin graft donor areas

Author details

Madhuri A. Gore*, Kabeer Umakumar and Sandhya P. Iyer

*Address all correspondence to: drmadhuri@hotmail.com

Department of General Surgery LTMGH & LTMMC, Sion, Mumbai

References

[1] Banana Leaf dressing for skin graft donor areas ; Gore M A, Akolekar D; Burns 2003 (29): 483 – 486

[2] Managing burns in India; focusing on newer strategies; Ahuja RB; Indian J. Burns 1995; 3:1

[3] Skin grafting – Article by Donald Grenade MD; www.emedicine.com/dem/top867(last update sept. 19,2006)

[4] Comparison of calcium sodium alginate and porcine xenograft (E-Zderm) in the healing of STSG donor sites; Vanstralen P; Burns 1992 (18), 145 – 48.

[5] Which dressing for STSG donor site? ; Feldman L; Ann plast Surg. 1991 (27): 288 – 91 .

[6] Story of plastic surgery; Davis JS ; Ann Surg; 1941 (113) 651 – 56.

[7] A prospective trial comparing biofane, duoderm and xeroderm for STSG donor site; Feldman D, Rogers A, Karpinski R; Surg gynae obst. 1991 (173) : 1-5.

[8] How to dress STSG donor sites ? A prospective, randomized study of four dressings ; Persson K, Salemark L; Scand J Plast Reconstr Surg Hand Surg. 2000 March (34-1): 55-9

[9] A randomized prospective trial comparing a hydrophilic polyurethane absorbent foam dressing with a petrolatum gauze dressing; Weber RS, Hankins P, Limitone F,. Callender D, Frankenthaler R.M, Wolf P, Goepfert H; Arch Otogaryngoal Head Neck Surg, 1995 Oct.; 121(10) :1145 – 49

[10] A comparison of calcium alginate and scarlet red dressings in the healing of STSG donor sites, Lawrence JE, Blake GB; Br J Plast Surg., 1992 Aug- Sept; 45 (6): 488.

[11] Use of honey as an adjunct in the healing of STSG donor site; Misir liogly A, Erogly S, Karacaoglan N, Akan M, Akoz T, Yildeirm S, Dermatolog Surg; 2003 Feb; 29 (2): 168 – 72 .

[12] Topical Phenytoin in the treatment of STSG donor sites : A comparative study with polyurethane membrane drape and conventional dressing; Yadav J.K., Singhvi AM, Kumar N, Garg S; Burns Aug 1993; 19(4): 306 – 10

[13] Hydrocolloid dressings in small and medium STSG donor sites?, Santamaria AB, Oroz J. Pelay M.I. , Castro J.A., Escudero F; Annals of MBC June 1992; 5:2

[14] Collagen dressing in the management of STSG donor sites; P. Halankar, D. Cunha – Gomes, C Chaudhari; Bombay Hosp J, 2005 Apr (5): 110 -12

[15] Comparison of the effect of a collagen dressing and a polyurethane dressing on the healing of STSG donor sites; Horch RE, Stark GB; Scan J Plast Reconstr Surg Hand Surg 1998 Dec; 32 (4): 407 – 13.

Chapter 8

Use of Skin Grafts in Free Flap Reconstruction

Anya Li, Mark K. Wax and Tamer Ghanem

Additional information is available at the end of the chapter

http://dx.doi.org/10.5772/53305

1. Introduction

Free flap reconstruction often results in a composite defect at the donor site. Many of these defects can be closed primarily (scapular free flaps, rectus abdominis free flap, and anterolateral thigh free flaps). However, some donor sites, such as fibular free flaps and radial forearm free flap, are particularly difficult to close primarily and require the use of skin grafts for coverage of the underlying muscle and tendon. There are several options available for obtaining material to cover the donor site defect.

1. Split thickness skin grafts harvested from a different anatomical site than free flap donor site
2. Split thickness skin graft harvested from the free flap donor site
3. Full thickness skin grafts harvested from a site adjacent to free flap donor site

Coverage with a skin graft compared to primary closure has not been shown to have increased complication rates [1] and decreases wound tension leading to less wound contracture, or worst yet, compartment syndrome [2]. We will discuss the different options for closure of free flap donor sites with skin grafts and the techniques to employ these options in the clinical practice.

2. Split thickness skin graft from a different anatomical site

The most common soft tissue free flap donor sites used in reconstructive surgery that require adjunctive closure techniques are the radial forearm and fibular free flap donor sites.

Preoperative considerations for taking a split thickness skin graft from a different anatomical site to close the defect include:

1. Skin thickness at the donor site. Elderly patients have thinner skin which can make taking a split thickness skin graft from certain areas difficult.
2. Need for a skin graft versus primary closure.

Advantages include:

1. Larger sized skin graft can be taken to account for shrinkage of the skin graft and decreased need for meshing.
2. Thicker skin graft can also be harvested from anatomical sites with thicker skin for better cosmetic outcomes i.e. better color retention and less contraction with healing.
3. Reduces free flap donor site wound tension closure.

Disadvantages include:

1. Color and hair mismatch
2. Increased morbidity from second donor site – pain, infection, wound care
3. Cosmetic defect at skin graft donor site
4. More wound care needed at free flap site compared to primary closure

We recommend harvesting the skin graft from an anatomical location that can be easily concealed such as the anterior or medial thigh, hip, or buttocks. The need for assistance in postoperative wound care can make the buttocks less advantageous. Special considerations for covering a free flap donor site include the underlying tissue and the thickness of the skin graft. Some free flap donor sites are left with minimally vitalized structures such as tendons and thicker skin grafts have higher metabolic demands. Thicker skin grafts placed over tendons may result in graft failure at those areas.

Harvest of the skin graft should be performed in a standard fashion.

1. First the patient should be positioned so the skin graft donor site is easily accessible to the surgeon.
2. The skin should be prepped initially with betadine and residual betadine should be washed off so the skin is clean. DuraPrep (3M, St Paul, MN) should not be used because it is difficult to remove.
3. Mineral oil should be applied liberally to the skin surface to facilitate movement of the dermatome.
4. An appropriately sized blade should be chosen (2, 3, or 4 inches) and a powered dermatome should be use (e.g. Zimmer, Warsaw, IN). The blade should be adjusted to the desired thickness, generally between 0.014 and 0.018 inches.
5. Position the blade at one end of the donor site and engage the skin with the dermatome at a 90-degree angle. Once engaged, shift to a 30 to 40-degree angle to the skin with an assistant using tongue depressors to keep the skin taught as the dermatome is advanced with constant downward pressure to harvest the skin graft in one piece.

6. Once the appropriately sized skin graft has been harvested, angle the blade up to terminate the harvest and carefully lift the skin graft away.

7. Punctate bleeding may be stopped with a combination of pressure, thrombin, and epinephrine soaked gauze. The donor site may be dressed with fibrin glue and covered with a tegaderm. The skin graft should be placed in saline until transfer to site for coverage.

While the skin graft may be harvested at the time of free flap resection, an alternative is delayed harvest with interval placement of Integra artificial dermis (Integra Lifesicences Corp, Plainsborough, NJ). Integra is a two layered product with a silicone outer layer that acts as a barrier for infection, heat, and moisture loss. The second layer is a matrix of cross-linked fibers that acts as a scaffold for dermal regeneration. An alternative is Oasis wound matrix (Cook Biotec Inc, West Lafayette, IN) which is an absorbable matrix derived from porcine intestinal sub mucosa. The matrix material is cut to a size to completely cover the defect. If Integra is used, the silicone layer is removed 2-3 weeks later once the dermis has regenerated. Then an epidermal layer is applied.

Advantages of using an absorbable matrix include allowing the patient to heal first from their primary resection and free flap before adding on another surgical site. Integra can allow a neodermis to form over minimally vitalized structures such as tendon to improve coverage and decrease risk of tendon exposure. It can also enhance cosmesis with better skin mobility after application of the epidermal layer or split thickness skin graft [3].

3. Split thickness skin graft from free flap donor site

The main advantage of harvesting the skin graft from the flap skin paddle is to avoid the donor site morbidity of an additional donor site. Studies have not shown any difference in morbidity of the free flap site when closing with a skin graft taken from the myo/osteocutaneous skin paddle versus from a different anatomical site. [4, 5].

Advantages:

1. Elimination of second skin graft donor site and associated morbidity which include potential for infection and pain which is often worse than the primary surgical site, and a second scar.

2. Reduction in free flap donor site wound tension closure.

Disadvantages:

1. Contraction of skin graft often requiring meshing and/or purse string suture technique

2. More wound care needed compared to primary closure

3. Risk of tendon exposure in certain areas such as radial forearm or fibula skin paddle

Harvest of the skin graft should be performed in the same fashion as described above with harvest from a separate donor site.

1. The skin graft should be harvested over the area in approximately the same size as the skin paddle that is to be harvested with the free flap (Figure 1).

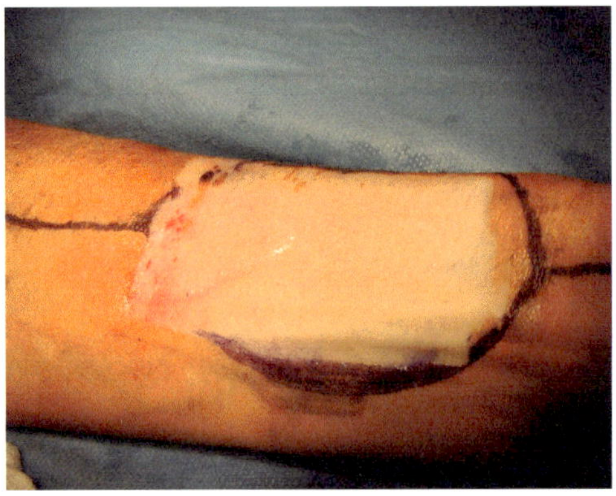

Figure 1. Split thickness skin graft taken from the flap site on the forearm.

2. The skin graft should be preserved in saline while the free flap is harvested. Once it is ready to fill the donor site, the skin graft should be measured and determined if meshing is needed. A 1:1.5 meshing grid is often adequate.

3. To reduce the wound bed surface area, a purse string suture technique may be employed (Figure 2). This technique is able to reduce the defect area by as much as 44.5% [6]. An absorbable suture such as 3-0 Vicryl (Ethicon Inc, Somerville, NJ) can be run in a subcuticular fashion along the periphery of the defect. The suture should be pulled taught so the circumference of the defect is reduced.

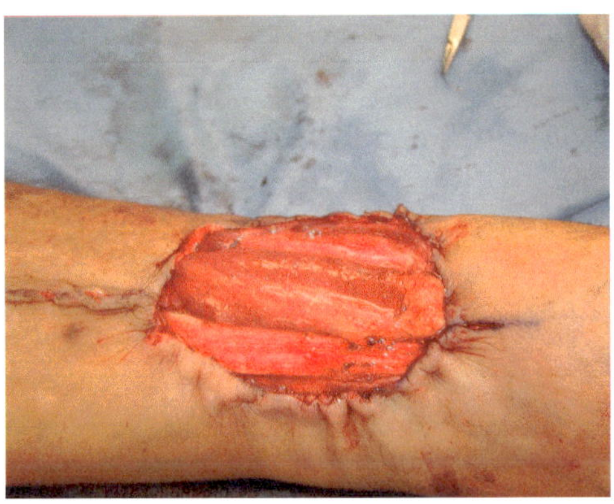

Figure 2. Purse string suture technique.

4. The meshed or non-meshed skin graft is then sewn in place to cover the donor site. If it is not meshed, small ventilation holes must be added in the graft to prevent fluid accumulation underneath the graft. (Figure 3a and 3b) Figure 4 shows a fully healed radial forearm donor site.

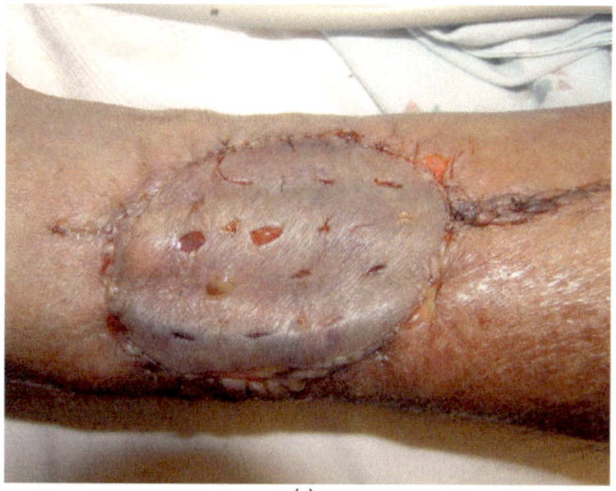

(a)

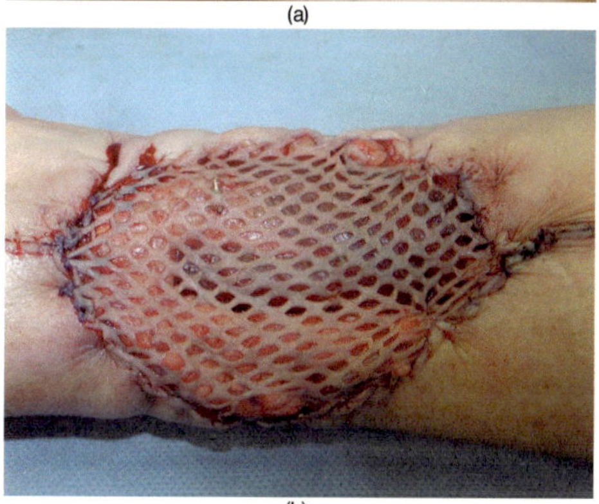

(b)

Figure 3. (a) Closure of donor site defect with non-meshed skin graft and purse string suture technique. (b) Closure of donor site defect with meshed skin graft and purse string suture technique.

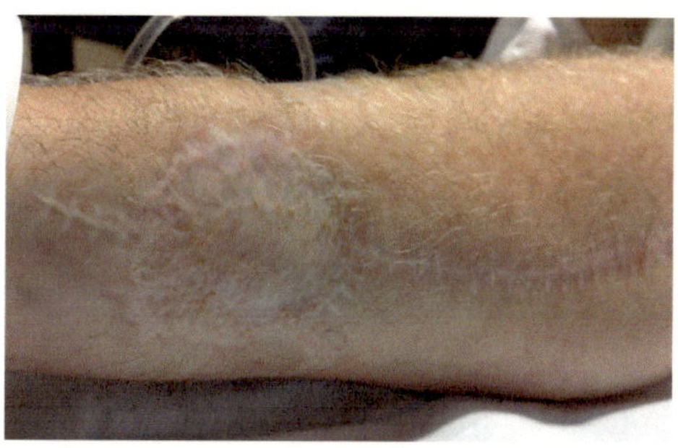

Figure 4. Fully healed radial forearm free flap donor site after purse string suture and meshed skin graft.

An alternative to fully elevating the skin graft is leaving one side hinged [7]. This decreases the amount of contracture, curling, scarring along the hinge site, and disruption of the graft. Additionally, it also maintains the orientation of the skin graft.

Special considerations include the thickness of the donor site. Often the elderly have thin skin which makes harvest from certain areas of the body such as the forearm challenging. Skin thickness stays relatively constant until about the 7th decade of life when it dimishes and came make skin grafts 0.015 inches in thickness or greater difficult to harvest in one piece [8].

4. Adjacent full thickness skin graft [9]

Preoperative considerations for using adjacent full thickness skin graft for coverage include the size of the defect. Because the skin graft will be taken from skin adjacent to the incision relating to the vascular pedicle, the laxity of the skin and circumference of the arm in relation to the donor defect must be measured. Skin that is not lax enough with a large donor defect to cover will result in circumferential skin tension around a limb and could result in compartment syndrome.

Advantages:

1. Better cosmesis with full thickness skin graft closure
2. Elimination of second skin graft donor site
3. Reduction in free flap donor site wound tension closure.

Disadvantages:

1. Only small defects can be covered
2. Full thickness skin graft donor site may have high tension with closure
3. Adjunctive closure techniques such as purse string suture may be necessary for coverage of the defect
4. More wound care needed compared to primary closure

Technique:

1. The donor defect must be measured and divided into 4 right triangles (Figure 5 – yellow area).
2. Each right triangle will correspond to one half of one side of the incision corresponding to the vascular pedicle (Figure 5 – red and blue areas).
3. The red and blue areas in Figure 5 are then harvested as full thickness skin grafts and divided in half to yield 4 right triangles which are then used to close the defect corresponding to the yellow area in Figure 5. A purse string suture technique may be used to decrease the defect size and decrease the amount of skin harvested.

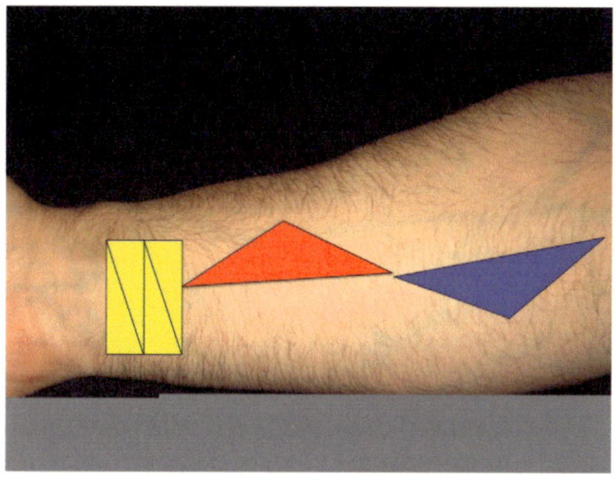

Figure 5. Schematic of full thickness skin grafts taken from skin adjacent to the incision for the vascular pedicle.

5. Conclusion

There are a variety of methods to close free flap donor sites including primary closure, full thickness, and split thickness skin grafts. None of these techniques have increased morbidity to the free flap donor site and the use of skin grafts help to decrease wound tension closure compared to primary closure. The main difference between the various methods is the variation in cosmetic outcome. This can be mitigated with purse string sutures, thicker skin grafts, and use of an artificial wound matrix.

Author details

Anya Li[1*], Mark K. Wax[2] and Tamer Ghanem[1]

*Address all correspondence to: ali1@hfhs.org

1 Department of Otolaryngology, Henry Ford Hospital, Detroit, MI, USA

2 Department of Otolaryngology, Oregon Heath Sciences, Portland, OR, USA

References

[1] Momoh AO, Yu P, Skoracki RJ, Liu S, Feng L, Hanasono MM. A Prospective Cohort Study of Fibula Free Flap Donor-Site Morbidity in 157 Consecutive Patients. Plast. Reconstr. Surg. 128(3): 714-720, 2011.

[2] Shindo M, Fong B, Funk G, et al. The fibula osteocutaneous flap in head and neck reconstruction: a critical evaluation of donor site morbidity. Arch Otolaryngol Head Neck Surg 2000;126:1467–72.

[3] Murray RC, Gordin EA, K Saigal K, Levelnthal D, Krein H, Heffelfinger RN. Reconstruction of the radial forearm free flap donor site using Integra artificial dermis. Microsurgery 31:104–108, 2011.

[4] Ghanem TA, Wax MK. A novel split–thickness skin graft donor site: the radial skin paddle. Otolaryngol Head Neck Surg. 2009;141(3):390-394.

[5] Kim PD, Fleck T, Heffelfinger R, Blackwell KE. Avoiding secondary skin graft donor site morbidity in the fibula free flap harvest. Arch Otolaryngol Head Neck Surg. 2008;134(12):1324-1327.

[6] Winslow CP, Vu KC, Mackenzie D, et al. Purse string suture closure of radial forearm fasciocutaneous donor sites. Laryngoscope 2000; 110:1815– 8.

[7] Boahene K, Richmon J, Byrne P, Ishii L. Hinged Forearm Split-Thickness Skin Graft for Radial Artery Fasciocutaneous Flap Donor Site Repair. Arch Facial Plast Surg. 2011;13(6):392-394

[8] de Rigal J, Escoffier C, Querleux B, Faivre B, Agache P, Leveque JL. Assessment of aging of the human skin by in vivo ultrasonic imaging. J Invest Dermatol. 1989;93(5): 621-625.

[9] González-García R, Ruiz-Laza L, Manzano D, Monje F. Combined local triangular full-thickness skin graft for the closure of the radial forearm free flap donor site: a new technique. Plast Reconstr Surg. 2010;125(2):85e-86e.